Praise for
HEALTH BLISS: 50 Revitalizing NatureFoods & Lifestyle Choices to Promote Vibrant Health

"HEALTH BLISS is a vitally important treasure trove of knowledge wrapped up in an easy-to-read, easy-to-understand package. Susan tells you how to select, prepare, and store 50 familiar—but nutritionally rich—foods and how to use them medicinally. This book is worth buying for the delicious Green Smoothie recipes alone! Like her earlier book The Healing Power of NATUREFOODS, this new book is a must-read for everyone interested in vibrant physical, mental, and spiritual health."

— **Neal Barnard, M.D.,**
founder and president, Physicians Committee for
Responsible Medicine; the author of
Dr. Neal Barnard's Program for Reversing Diabetes

"After reading HEALTH BLISS, your thinking about food will be transformed. Dr. Jones has diligently searched the medical and scientific literature to identify the most important healing foods, and she shares the fruits of her efforts in this thoroughly understandable and entertaining book. You will be amazed at how much control you can have over your health simply by choosing the proper foods!"

— **Brian S. Boxer Wachler, M.D.,**
director, Boxer Wachler Vision Institute, Beverly Hills, California

"Susan's new book, HEALTH BLISS, will help you take the important first steps toward optimal health. She teaches you why it's so vitally important to eat nutrient-rich foods if you wish to achieve superior nutrition and enjoy the accompanying health benefits. If you are new to healthful eating, this is an excellent introduction to good diet and beyond."

— **Joel Fuhrman, M.D.,**
the author of *Eat to Live*

"Susan's frequent appearances on my radio shows are always
well received, and because of her popularity and esteemed expertise
in holistic health, I often invite her to fill in for me as the host when I'm away.
Gratefully, I now have another superb book of hers to recommend
to my listeners, friends, and family. HEALTH BLISS *presents*
a compelling road map through the health highways of life.
It offers a fresh approach and a powerful message for anyone
who desires to experience optimal health, unlimited joy, and a peaceful life.
Woven into this very insightful story of how foods affect our bodies
are countless practical health and balanced-living principles that can
change your life forever! Her 'Green Smoothie' recipes are now a part of my daily
nutrition program. If we all lived as Susan suggests, America could close most
of its hospitals and jails and become a nation in health and peace with itself rather
than an environment of stress, unhappiness, and ailments—obesity, diabetes,
heart disease, cancer, and arthritis, just to name a few. Susan's latest book is
definitely worth reading over and over again; it will engage your mind, inspire
your heart, and change your life for the better, just as it has for me."

— **Nick Lawrence,**
radio/TV talk-show host

❦ ❦ ❦

"You and I have the power, the right, and the freedom
to choose for ourselves how to best live our lives.
There is never a choice-less moment. The way we evolve
and transform ourselves is through our choices."

— from *You Are Your Choices,* by **Alexandra Stoddard**

❋ ❋ ❋

HEALTH BLISS

50 Revitalizing NatureFoods

&

Lifestyle Choices to Promote Vibrant Health

Susan Smith Jones, Ph.D.

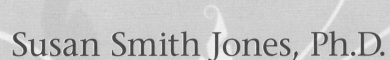

HAY HOUSE, INC.
Carlsbad, California • New York City
London • Sydney • Johannesburg
Vancouver • Hong Kong • New Delhi

Published and distributed in the United States by: Hay House, Inc.: www.hayhouse.com •
Published and distributed in Australia by: Hay House Australia Pty. Ltd.: www.hayhouse.com.au
• *Published and distributed in the United Kingdom by:* Hay House UK, Ltd.: www.hayhouse.co.uk
• *Published and distributed in the Republic of South Africa by:* Hay House SA (Pty), Ltd.: www.
hayhouse.co.za • *Distributed in Canada by:* Raincoast: www.raincoast.com • *Published in India
by:* Hay House Publishers India: www.hayhouse.co.in

Editorial supervision: Jill Kramer   •   *Design:* Charles McStravick

Library of Congress Cataloging-in-Publication Data

Jones, Susan Smith.
  Health bliss : 50 revitalizing superfoods & lifestyle choices to promote vibrant health / Susan Smith Jones. -- 1st ed.
     p. cm.
  "Volume II."
  Sequel to: The healing power of naturefoods. 2006.
  ISBN-13: 978-1-4019-1241-3 (tradepaper) 1. Functional foods. 2. Natural foods. I. Jones, Susan Smith- Healing power of naturefoods. II. Title.
  QP144.F85J662 2007
  613.2--dc22   2007047015

ISBN: 978-1-4019-1241-3

11 10 09 08   4 3 2 1
1st edition, June 2008

This book is gratefully dedicated to Louise L. Hay—
my mentor, my friend, and my earth angel.
Without your loving support and encouragement,
this book would not have been written.
Thank you for showing me, by example,
how to dream BIG, live fully,
and celebrate life.

It's also lovingly dedicated to God and Christ
for gracing my life with unlimited blessings,
priceless lessons, infinite possibilities,
and everlasting love.

And finally my gratitude goes to you, the reader.
I salute your great adventure.
May you be well nourished by healthful foods,
a grateful heart, and lots of love.

❋ ❋ ❋

MENU

PART I: HORS D'OEUVRES

    Foreword 3

    Introduction 7

    10 Surefire Steps to Create an Abundantly Healthy Life 13

    A Fresh Approach to Healthful Eating & Living 21

PART II: ENTRÉES

    50 NatureFoods: Part I 33

        Açai Berries 37

        Aloe Vera 39

        Apricots 41

        Artichokes 42

        Arugula 44

        Barley Grass 44

        Berries 46

        Burdock Root 48

        Cabbage 49

        Cauliflower 51

        Cherimoya 52

        Cherries 53

        Chicory 55

        Chlorella 55

        Chlorophyll 57

        Collards 58

        Corn 59

        Daikon 61

        Dandelion 62

        Dark Chocolate 63

        Dates 65

        Evening Primrose 66

        Fennel 68

        Fermented Foods 69

        Flower Blossoms 71

PART III: INTERMISSION

The Healing Power of . . .

Deep Breathing 77

Neti: Nasal Cleansing 83

Sleep 89

A Healthy Metabolism 95

Beautiful Skin 103

Sweating & Saunas 111

Exercise 117

Silence & Solitude 121

Love 127

Salubrious Green Smoothies 129

PART IV: MORE ENTRÉES

50 NatureFoods: Part II 139

Go Green 139

Grapes & Raisins 142

Green Beans 143

Herbs & Spices 144

Jicama 148

Lavender 149

Lentils 150

Limes 151

Mango 152

Meyer Lemon 152

Millet 153

Miso 155

Papaya 155

Peppermint 156

Pineapple 157

Plums & Prunes 159

Pumpkin & Pumpkin Seeds 160

Quinoa 162

Sea Salt 163
Squash 164
Turnips 165
Wakame 167
Watercress 168
Wheatgrass 169
Yellow Split Peas 170

PART V: Radiant Health at a Glance

Radiant Health at a Glance Table 173

PART VI: Recipes

Salubrious Green Smoothie Recipes 179

PART VII: Motivational Tools

Affirmations 199
21-Day Agreement 203

Afterword 207
Gratitude 211
Resources
    Recommended Reading & Websites 213
    Some of My Favorite Health-Promoting Products 217
    Books & Audio Programs by Susan Smith Jones 219
Index 223
About the Author 235

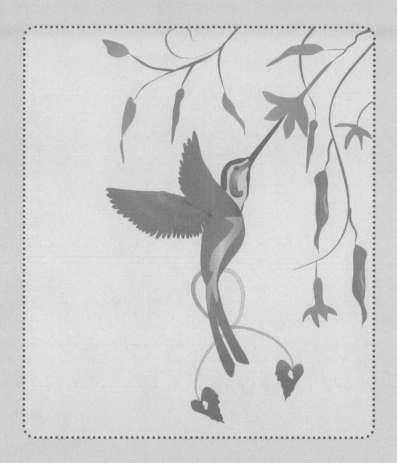

PART I

HORS D'OEUVRES

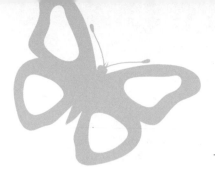

FOREWORD

"I've watched Susan's star rise for many years.
I am so proud to say that she is now a Hay House author.
Her work with NatureFoods is legendary."

— LOUISE L. HAY

I'm a big admirer of holistic health consultant and author Susan Smith Jones. I call her the "NatureFoods Lady" because she has been my source of inspiration and information about the wonderful world of NatureFoods for as long as I can remember. After many years of reading her books, I finally asked if she would like to be a Hay House author. Nothing brings me greater joy than to be part of bringing an individual author's work to a wider audience.

Just like Susan, I'm a big fan of NatureFoods—foods rich in nutrients and antioxidants that promote health, healing, and vitality, no matter what your age. Susan is a baby boomer, and you should see how vibrantly young and alive she looks—she's living proof that her advice *really works*. I urge you to take her wise counsel to heart.

There are many ways to change your life. Working with my ideas on "changing your thoughts to change your life" isn't the only option. There's a spiritual approach, there's the mental approach, and there's the physical approach, as Susan details in this superb book. When you clean your house, it doesn't really matter which room you start in. Just begin in the area that appeals to you most, and the others will happen almost by themselves.

The same applies to healing your body. I usually give very little nutritional advice (unless someone asks) because I've discovered that different methods work for different people. But Susan's commonsense approach to healthful eating and living is really advantageous for everyone because her basic philosophy is simple and efficacious: *"Choose to eat your foods as close to the way nature made them as possible."* Because of Susan, I've adopted a similar, simple approach to eating: If it grows, eat it. If it doesn't grow, don't eat it.

Be conscious of your eating, the way Susan suggests. It's like paying attention to your thoughts. You can learn to listen to your body and the signals you get when you eat in different ways. Cleaning the mental house after a lifetime of indulging in negative thoughts is a bit like going on a good nutrition program after decades of indulging in junk foods. They both can create healing crises. As you begin to change your physical diet, the body starts to throw off the accumulations of toxic residue; and as this happens, you can feel rather rotten for a day or two. So it is when you make a decision to change your thought patterns—your circumstances can seem worse for a while.

Recall for a moment the end of a Thanksgiving dinner. The food is eaten, and it's time to clean the turkey pan. The interior is all burnt and crusty, so you pour in hot water and soap and let it soak for a while. Then you begin to scrape it, and you really have a mess. It looks worse than ever, but if you just keep scrubbing away, soon you'll have a pan as good as new.

It's the same with cleaning up a dried-on mental pattern. When we soak it with new ideas, all the good comes to the surface for us to look at. Just keep doing the affirmations that Susan offers you in this book, and soon you'll have completely cleared an old limitation.

Susan's premise in this informative book is: Think health, whole foods, and simple lifestyle choices. While we all know that healthful eating is one of the main keys to a long life, few of us understand which specific foods and other lifestyle choices can help protect the body and cultivate optimal well-being. Susan's three-book health series for Hay House, *The Healing Power of NatureFoods, Health Bliss,* and *Recipes for Health Bliss: Using NatureFoods to Rejuvenate Your Body & Life* (available from Hay House, June 2009), combines the latest research on the NatureFoods that prevent the most common age-related illnesses with essential information on the healing power of raw foods; exercise; sleep; dry skin brushing; deep breathing; boosting metabolism; pH balance; water; and a positive, grateful attitude. She offers you a comprehensive understanding of the amazing health potential of plant-based foods and shows you how to enjoy a level of health and vitality you never dreamed possible.

This new book will teach you how to create the youthful vigor, well-being, energy, and peace you desire and deserve. What's more, as a culinary-savvy educator and private natural-foods chef, Susan will inspire you with simple ways to make healthful meals; she provides a sampling of colorful recipes that are as easy to prepare as they are enjoyable to eat.

You're in for a treat as you read and savor every page of this book.

— Louise L. Hay

"At times our own light goes out and is
rekindled by a spark from another person.
Think of those, with deep gratitude,
who have lighted the flame within us."

— ALBERT SCHWEITZER

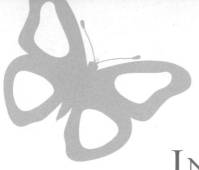

INTRODUCTION

*"The wise man should consider that
health is the greatest of human blessings.
Let food be your medicine and medicine be your food."*

— HIPPOCRATES

My reason for creating this book is really quite simple: I have a passion for writing—for sharing my thoughts, experiences, and research on being healthy, happy, and fully alive—and a desire to help make a positive difference in people's lives. As you read, I want you to feel as though we're sitting across from each other, and I'm talking to you personally. I already know that we have lots in common, since you've chosen to read about how to eat and live healthfully and how to be the very best you can be.

This book builds upon and expands the principles I described in *The Healing Power of NatureFoods: 50 Revitalizing SuperFoods & Lifestyle Choices to Promote Vibrant Health.* As a health researcher, writer, teacher, lecturer, counselor, and lifestyle coach for 35 years, I've learned that the secrets to joy and fulfillment in this life are found in the study and practice of holistic health, optimal nutrition, and balanced living. My friends and clients call me "the NatureFoods Lady" and "the Nature Girl" because I always look to nature for answers to life's ongoing health questions.

If you're new to my work, here's my health philosophy in a nutshell, beautifully described by Ralph Waldo Emerson: *"Health is our greatest wealth."* If you think about this sage advice, I'm sure you'll agree. Fortunately, regardless of your age, current level of well-being, and present diet or living habits, you can choose differently at any moment. Your new, better choices will lead to a healthier and happier life than you ever thought possible.

If you're a "baby boomer" like I am, keep in mind that changes that were once labeled milestones of growing older—such as high blood pressure, fragile bones, significant memory loss, wrinkles, reduced vision, and lack of energy and libido—are no longer considered inevitable. The diet and lifestyle choices I recommend in this book (and practice myself) will help you look and feel vibrantly alive at any age. I feel as young and exuberant as I ever did—and you can, too!

Your level of health, right this moment, is the result of the countless decisions you've made regarding your diet, exercise, thought processes, beliefs, and expectations. Undoubtedly, many of these choices have been poor ones, but you can use your past mistakes and learn from them. However, you must start with a commitment. Specifically, are you willing to make a commitment to your health?

Such dedication begins with appreciating, respecting, and loving your magnificent body. *One of the most important things you can learn in life is to appreciate yourself. As you open your heart to your own self-worth and to the divine essence of all humanity, you access the most powerful healer of all, the healing power of love.* And the human body is, indeed, a miracle of love's creation. The more I study our physical structure, the more I am amazed and in awe at how beautifully it is designed. Clearly, it's a fantastic creation that deserves reverence and respect.

Your body is a remarkable feedback machine. If you listen, you'll discover that it actually talks to you. When you get a headache, for instance, your physical self is trying to tell you something. Receive its signals with health, balance, and peace as your goals. The key here is your willingness to listen and act. Start today to tune in more.

Most people think that the way to handle a headache is to reach for a bottle of aspirin. They believe that it's normal to experience such discomfort, but they're mistaken. While headaches (and the countless other aches and pains that people experience) are certainly common, health is the truly normal state. Disease is an aberration, caused either by harm you've done to yourself or that others have done to you.

Collectively, Americans have been making some very poor choices. Just look at all of the commercials on television and the advertisements in magazines and newspapers. Whatever you're suffering from—headache, constipation, sleepless nights, diarrhea, indigestion, skin rashes, high blood pressure, impotency . . . fill in the blank—the advertisers have a miracle pill, powder, or potion for you. We've come to believe that things outside ourselves are the keys to health and well-being.

We've become a self-medicating society because we don't really understand how beautifully robust the human body is. Each of us needs to be reminded that we're magnificently equipped to meet life's problems when supplied with the simple and easily obtainable requisites of health.

Choose to Make Positive Changes

I have some astonishing news for you: It's normal to be able to go to sleep at night without taking a pill. It's normal not to have headaches, sinus problems, hemorrhoids, constipation, and shaky hands. It's normal to be well. We just need to *stop doing the things that cause the problems in the first place.* When you live more from inner guidance, closer to nature, you can enrich the quality of your life and the life on this planet. It's simply a matter of choice. And it all begins, as mentioned previously, with appreciating, respecting, and taking loving care of your body. The body reflects the mind, and the mind reflects the spirit, so choosing to make positive changes with your miraculous body is a good place to start.

This book focuses primarily on how to take the best care of your body—starting today—by choosing to eat healthful foods and taking steps to improve a variety of other necessary habits. You see, it's really not about making major lifestyle or dietary changes; rather, it's about making simple, *effective* choices. What you eat, how much you move or sleep, what you think, how you deal with stress, how much water you drink, how many bad habits you can discard, and how much your social relationships support you—these factors have a profound effect on health, longevity, and quality of life.

Of the many positive steps you can take, three are eminently under your control: what you eat, how much you move (physical activity), and what you think about. You have the ability to change all of these at any time. For example, you're the one who decides what you eat or drink; nobody, I hope, shoves the food down your throat. If you want to be vibrantly healthy, free from disease, and filled with energy and vitality, start upgrading.

Most people are digging their graves with their knives and forks each and every day. While your diet is only one of the essential ingredients of vibrant health, it's a big one. Think about it this way: Your body is composed of more than 70 trillion cells. Envision each cell as a little engine. Some of them work in unison and some independently, and they're all on the job 24/7. In order for the engines to work right, they require specific fuels. If one is given the wrong type, it won't be able to perform to maximum capacity. If the fuel is of a poor grade, the engine may sputter and hesitate, creating a loss of power. If it isn't given any of what it needs, it will stop.

Much of the fuel for our cells comes directly from the things we eat. Food contains nutrients in the form of vitamins, minerals, water, carbohydrates, fats, proteins, and enzymes. Just as a car requires different forms of energy for the brakes, transmission, and battery to run smoothly, our cells require various types and amounts of nutrients, depending on their location and function in the body. These nutrients allow us to sustain life by providing our cells with the basic materials they need to carry on. Each nutrient we ingest differs in form, function, and amount needed; however, all of them are vital. They're involved in every bodily process, whether it be combating infection, providing energy, or promoting tissue repair, but their common goal is to keep us going. Although eating has been woven into many cultural and religious practices, its essential purpose is survival.

A fundamental problem for most people is eating too much low-nutrient food. These poor choices deprive your body of the nutrients you need. When you do this for a long enough period of time, you get sick because normal functions are impaired. Even if you aren't obviously sick, you may not necessarily be healthy. It simply may be that you aren't yet exhibiting any overt symptoms of illness. Unlike a car engine, which immediately malfunctions if you put water into the gasoline tank, the human body has tremendous resilience and often camouflages the repercussions of unhealthful fuel choices. By understanding the principles of holistic nutrition and knowing what nutrients you need and what foods contain them, you can improve the state of your health, stave off disease, and maintain the harmonious balance that nature intended.

Trying to Buy Health

One of the most sobering national statistics is that the U.S. spent $1.5 trillion on disease care last year, more per capita than any other nation in the world. But we're nowhere near the top of the list when it comes to health. Despite our high-tech therapies, we're lagging behind all of the other industrialized nations and a number of developing countries, as well. How can this be?

One big reason is that there are huge food and medical industries working hard to convince us that what we eat has little or no effect on our health. We're told by industry apologists that any combination of low-nutrient, processed, chemicalized "foods" will meet our needs as long as we take plenty of vitamins, heartburn medicine, headache pills, and other remedies. By contrast, scientists tell us that by the year 2015, more than 75 percent of all Americans will be obese (with all of the diseases that accompany this condition). You don't need to be a Nobel Prize winner to understand that Western medicine needs to rethink how it views health and well-being, and that changes need to be made *now*.

Eating for Optimal Health

As study after study has shown, a high-nutrient, plant-based diet is a prerequisite for optimal health. That's why half of this book is devoted to identifying 50 of the most healthful foods—what I refer to as NatureFoods—and describing their benefits. I've also included some easy-to-prepare recipes that just happen to be as delicious as they are nutritious. Add these NatureFoods and recipes to those you'll find in my book *The Healing Power of NatureFoods,* and you'll have 100 of the best ingredients to help reduce your risks of heart disease, hypertension, diabetes, obesity, Alzheimer's, arthritis, common forms of cancer, premature aging, vision problems, and mental dysfunction. I'll also describe the ones that help accelerate fat loss, increase your energy level and joie de vivre, and empower you to achieve control over your life.

I list the foods in alphabetical order. Each one is backed by extensive research and my personal experience of teaching nutrition and healthful food-preparation classes (cooked and live-food cuisine) for more than 35 years. Please note that while I am not a proponent of animal testing, I have mentioned a few such scientific studies in the book simply for reference.

As you'll discover, there's more to radiant well-being than a good diet. Other essential factors must be integrated into your life if you want to maximize your health potential. These include physical factors such as fresh air, plenty of rest and sleep, exercise, sunshine, internal and external cleanliness, and the avoidance of addictions. Also important are mental factors, such as a positive attitude; deep respect for life; high self-esteem; daily respites of solitude and silence; a sense of belonging; and an awareness and trust in your Higher Power, God, or whatever you choose to call this loving presence. I also encourage you to explore practices such as meditation, deep breathing, intentional profuse sweating (saunas), and body balancing.

I describe some of these topics in this book. For more in-depth information about these and other practices, please refer to my books and audio programs

BE HEALTHY~STAY BALANCED, Choose to Live Peacefully, Wired to Meditate, Choose to Live Fully, and *EVERYDAY HEALTH—Pure & Simple.*

I encourage you to make a commitment for 90 days—just one season, three months—and incorporate as many of my dietary and lifestyle suggestions as possible into your routine. In this short period of time, you'll look better than you have in years and also feel more youthful and empowered. In fact, if you make the commitment for 90 days, you can turn back the clock by at least a decade. That's right—you can look and feel ten years younger! What do you have to lose except some extra weight, aches and pains, ailments and diseases, and a negative attitude toward your body and your life? I know you can do it. I believe in you and salute your great adventure, and I hope to meet you in person somewhere along the way.

❋ ✻ ❋

10 Surefire Steps to Create an Abundantly Healthy Life

"Love yourself, heal your life."

— Louise L. Hay

One of the greatest truths of life is that it flows from the inside out. We're affected by what happens inside—our feelings and our thoughts—which, in turn, affect our emotions, the words we speak, and the actions we choose to take. What you feel or experience at any point in time is up to you. Change your thoughts, and you change your life.

Easier said than done, right? Well, in this section, I'll tell you the ten best ways I know to create abundant health and happiness and help you understand your inner world better so that you can create more success in your life. And a great place to start is with the important role of your mind in creating positive change.

Your mind is a powerful tool for bringing about beneficial change and success, but it isn't always your friend. Sometimes it's a less-than-willing partner; at points, it may actually undermine your good intentions. As an example, let's look at how your thoughts can make or break a new exercise program.

Everyone knows that exercise is of paramount importance in creating vibrant health. Perhaps you've taken up walking or jogging and promised yourself that you're going to hit the trail at least every other day. At first, you have a lot of motivation and meet your goals. But as the days spin by, your resolve starts to flag a bit. It seems that something always comes up that appears to be more important than exercise. Perhaps you need to be in the office early and can't take time for a morning run, or you might have to take one of your children somewhere and it prevents you from taking your afternoon walk. Maybe you stay out late one night, and an extra hour of sleep seems more inviting than a few laps in the pool.

Whatever circumstances you create (they rarely just *arise*), and no matter how legitimate they seem at the time, be aware that your mind is more than happy to help you create excuses so that you can slip back into familiar patterns. According to behavioral psychologists, *it takes 21 days of consistently repeating an activity before your mind accepts it as a habit.*

Here are the first three Surefire Steps you can take to ensure you'll stick with your new exercise program. (Later in the book, you'll find my list of 101 Reasons to Exercise, as well as a 21-Day Agreement form that you can use to help boost your motivation and keep you on purpose.)

1. Choose an exercise program that includes activities you honestly like to do. Ideally, you'll pick a variety—such as jogging, walking, hiking, bicycling, swimming, and weight lifting—that collectively work different muscle groups and offer diversity. Most important, select things that you won't dread doing a minimum of three times a week.

2. Create an exercise plan that seems easy to accomplish. You might, for instance, want to make an agreement with yourself that you'll spend 30 minutes jogging or walking (depending upon the way you feel) every day. Or you might agree to spend 15 minutes stretching or doing yoga each morning. Don't create a plan so difficult that it sets you up to fail, such as running or biking long distances every day. Your mind and body are designed to rebel against drastic changes, and their protests will see to it that you don't succeed.

3. Resolve to stay with your agreement every day for 21 days. If you skip a day in your program for some reason, you must begin the cycle over again. The reasoning behind this is simple: Because it takes 21 days to form a new habit, it will probably take that long for your mind and body to stop resisting the new pattern. Three weeks isn't a very long time, so if you find your mind coming up with excuses, you can regain control by reminding yourself that you only have to do it for 21 days.

If at the end of that time you still don't enjoy the activity or feel you aren't receiving any benefit, you always can reevaluate. What you'll almost surely find is that by the end of the trial period, you'll no longer mind doing the exercise. It will have become a normal part of your life. At this point, you'll be ready to incorporate a slightly more demanding fitness program, which I describe in detail in my books *Be Healthy~Stay Balanced* and *Choose to Live Fully.*

This 21-day process can be used in any area you choose, including changing your eating habits, drinking more water, getting more sleep, simplifying your home or office space (such as spending 15–20 minutes daily cleaning out and organizing drawers, closets, and cupboards), expanding your vocabulary, or establishing a meditation or prayer program.

Discipline & Commitment

Before we go on to the next seven steps, let's consider the importance of discipline and commitment. What you're probably realizing by now (and you'll understand it even better after reading the section of this book called *A Fresh Approach to Healthful Eating & Living*) is that discipline is an important part of creating your best, most abundant, and healthiest life. Discipline is a choice. If you're to achieve your highest potential, you must practice self-discipline in every aspect of your life. Success and fulfillment are available to you only if you learn to control your body, mind, and emotions.

Discipline, to me, means *the ability to carry out a resolution long after the mood has left you.* It also means doing what you say you're going to do—with courage, eagerness, and enthusiasm. If your attitude is positive, you'll get positive results. There's no way to achieve 100 percent success without putting in 100 percent effort.

With such resolution comes freedom and peace of mind. A disciplined person isn't at the mercy of external circumstances. Whereas someone without this quality is usually lazy, undirected, unhappy, or depressed, someone with it is in control of what she thinks, feels, says, and does. A disciplined mind creates a disciplined body, and from that comes an exhilarated mind. It's a powerful cycle.

This characteristic ignites your inherent inner power and helps create miracles in your life. Breakthroughs occur when people are willing to live out their vision and commitment and to honor their decisions. When you're committed, you allow nothing to deter you from reaching your goals. Discipline keeps you going even when you are not feeling motivated. You don't make excuses, and you follow through and do what you say that you're going to do.

Accountability

Make your word count; be responsible and accountable. How can you expect others to keep their obligations to you or have confidence that you'll keep yours unless you first show a firm commitment to yourself?

I welcome friendships with those to whom commitment, discipline, follow-through, and positive risk taking are integral to living and being. When I'm with those individuals, I feel empowered, inspired, motivated, and energized. I have very little patience or respect for people who don't honor their obligations; they can be a very big drain on my energy.

If you're ready for commitment and accountability—and prepared to create your best life—you'll arrange your personal circumstances so that your lifestyle totally supports your intentions. You'll do whatever it takes—including letting go of excess mental and emotional baggage and superfluous nonessentials—to consistently focus on what's important.

Self-mastery begins by recognizing your power and using it to bring your vision to life. Some years ago, I made a conscious choice to stop allowing myself to go where outside factors pushed and pulled me. Instead, I began to acknowledge that I could choose my responses and master my life. Since then, I've begun to use the power that I previously had been giving away to self-limiting beliefs. This moment—right now—can be a new beginning. You no longer need to repeat the past, worry about the future, or struggle through life as a victim of circumstance.

The next seven Surefire Steps will help boost your self-esteem and make life more of a celebration filled with success. As you'll see, while each of these tips is positive and nurturing, each one also requires a degree of discipline and commitment.

4. Take loving care of your body. Eat a variety of colorful, healthful foods and exercise regularly. Think of yourself as more than just flesh, bone, and tissue. Treat your physical self as the miracle it is, and honor it with love and respect.

Your body is self-repairing, self-healing, and self-maintaining. As a matter of course, it persistently marshals its forces in a tireless quest to achieve and maintain radiant health—which is your normal, natural state. When you're healthy, it automatically directs its efforts toward maintaining that condition. When you experience "dis-ease," it diligently strives to restore balance and health.

Unconditionally cherishing, appreciating, loving, respecting, and nurturing your body, no matter what your current shape or level of wellness, is one of the first steps to experiencing vibrant, radiant health and living your best life. Your body is your friend; give it tender, loving care. Although it may only be a temporary home for your spiritual being, it's still an incredible gift you must cherish and nurture daily.

5. Be grateful and count your blessings. Gratitude and appreciation are magnetic forces that draw blessings to you. This dynamic spiritual energy allows you to exert a powerful influence on your body and life. As Plato is said to have written, "A grateful mind is a great mind—it eventually attracts to itself every great thing."

Buy or create your own special gratitude journal. Every day, write down at least three things for which you're grateful. Remember, whatever you put your attention on expands and grows in your life.

Look at all of the positive aspects about your body and life, and write them down so you can see them all the time. Make a list of all the things for which you're grateful: your eyes, with which you see beauty; your hands, with which you touch and embrace; your children, spouse, and friends who support and love you unconditionally; your animal companions who bring you joy; the flowers in your yard; and the beautiful objects in your home that keep elegance in your daily life. *Think of your mind as a resplendent garden, and keep it beautiful and fragrant by cultivating a positive attitude and harvesting the bountiful rewards of gratitude.*

6. Be patient, trust, and act "as if." Everything happens in its proper time. Have confidence that unscheduled events in your life are your own form of spiritual direction and that everything will unfold for your highest good. Be patient with yourself, and choose to live one day at a time. Throughout the day, I affirm often: *I let go and let God (love, light, peace, Christ, or the like) guide my day (or take charge of this situation).*

When you feel frustrated that things aren't going as you planned and your dreams seem to be continually beyond your reach, don't give up. In fact, act as though your best life is yours right now, for on some level of your being, it is. If you want more peace in your life, you must choose to be peaceful; if you want more joy, be joyful. If you'd like more friends, you must first be a good companion to yourself and others. And if you wish for more prosperity, act and live as though you were experiencing your highest vision for yourself right now. In other words, acting "as if" will help you through many challenging times and will become a powerful bridge between you and possible channels of good in your life. It was Shakespeare who championed this sage advice in his immortal words in *Hamlet:* "Assume a virtue, if you have it not."

7. Let go of all criticism and judgments. Be loving and kind toward yourself. Harboring critical thoughts affects your body and health. When you let go of your self-criticisms and judgments of others, and instead choose to practice living with unconditional love and forgiveness, your authentic, beautiful self then reveals itself. So when you catch yourself coming to harsh conclusions, stop and think of something positive. Say your affirmations; count your blessings; and at least once each day, look in the mirror and take one minute to praise and support yourself. You deserve it. Later in this book is a sample list of 40 affirmations that you can use daily; and my books *Choose to Live Peacefully,* BE HEALTHY~STAY BALANCED, and *Choose to Live Fully* contain a plethora of information on affirmations, including their efficacy in creating what you want in life and how to use them.

8. Be of service to others. One of the fastest ways to feel better about yourself is to do something nice for another person. It could be as simple as giving someone a hug, cooking a meal for a sick neighbor, watching a friend's child so that she can have some quality time to herself, or sending a card saying "thank you." In giving to others, we give to ourselves. Find ways to volunteer. A ten-year study of 1,300 people in Michigan found that those who were active in organizations outside the home lived longer, healthier lives than those who weren't. Some scientists even speculate that volunteering produces a "helper's high," an exhilaration caused by the release of endorphins, the brain's own mood-elevating chemicals. I'm sure Albert Schweitzer would agree. He expressed the following sagacious thought: *"The only ones among you who will be really happy are those who have sought and found how to serve."*

9. Laugh as often as possible. This is one of the best ways I know to help mollify stress and enrich life. It's okay to laugh, even when times are tough. Toxic worry almost always entails a loss of perspective, and a sense of humor almost always restores it. For me, laughing often is truly the elixir of life.

Norman Cousins, the noted journalist and author, found a way to enrich his life even while in the midst of a life-threatening illness. He discovered that he was able to achieve two hours of pain-free living for every ten minutes he devoted to laughter. So he started watching old Marx Brothers comedies, *The Three Stooges, Candid Camera,* and other humorous TV shows and movies. Laughter became his best medicine.

Laughter—hearty belly laughs—produces chemicals in the brain that benefit body, mind, and emotions. And studies now disclose that laughing releases endorphins, which act as natural stress busters that aid most—and probably all—major systems of the body. A good laugh gives the heart muscles a workout; improves circulation; fills the lungs with oxygen-rich air; clears the respiratory passages; arouses alertness hormones that stimulate various tissues; helps relieve pain; alters the brain by diminishing tension in the central nervous system; and counteracts fear, anger, and depression, all of which are linked to physical illness and stress.

10. Live in the presence of loving thoughts. Nothing will transform your life more quickly than a consistent feeling of love in your heart. For the next 24 hours, maintain this emotion. Your entire life will change for the better, and you'll be enriched.

Be forewarned—staying in a loving state for 24 hours isn't very easy, but keep practicing and see how long you can go. When doing so, you're relinquishing all critical and judgmental thoughts about yourself and others and practicing continual forgiveness. Remember, you're always attracting back to yourself the equivalent of what you think, feel, say, and do. Strive to make your life about living in the presence of love and invite it to be your guide. A caring attitude and heart are magnets for unlimited blessings and miracles in your life and the lives of your loved ones.

❋ ❊ ❋

A Fresh Approach to Healthful Eating & Living

"The ordinary arts we practice every day at home
are of more importance to the soul than
their simplicity might suggest."

— Thomas Moore, poet

As I've said in the previous pages, your life involves millions of choices. Moment to moment, you're always choosing, and as life goes on, you become the results of what you pick. You are what you think, what you imagine, how you react, what you eat, how you move, what you say, what you feel, and what you expect in life. With that in mind, isn't it time to take full responsibility for the decisions you make? Start right now by acknowledging your immense power to create what you've always wanted—a healthy, fit body and a joyful, fulfilling, peaceful life.

Let's explore more closely the importance of day-to-day food choices and the need to reprogram and retrain your senses to choose empowerment and release self-limiting beliefs and habits. Your primary goal on this "aliveness" eating regimen is to get to the point where you're eating a sufficient amount of the highest-quality foods—including as many raw, living foods as possible. Euripides said, "Enough is abundance to the wise."

Loving Changes

Although it's important to choose healthful foods, don't become a fanatic about what you eat. Approach your new dietary habits with a loving heart. It's what you choose to eat on a daily basis that makes the biggest difference, not the occasional lapse. Be firm in your resolve to consume the highest-nutrient foods, but be kind and gentle with yourself during the initial implementation period. Worrying about every little bite that goes into your mouth is far more harmful in the long run than infrequent errors.

An important first step is to understand that the only way to ensure optimal nutrition is to eat a diet composed primarily of *whole plant foods, eaten in a form that's as close as possible to the way they come packaged by nature.* When you do so, you get all of the vitamins, minerals, enzymes, amino acids, natural sugars, fibers, and water that nature put into them, and you get them in the right proportions for efficient use by your body. Fresh, organic fruits, vegetables, whole grains, legumes, sprouts, nuts, and seeds (and if you still eat fish, the occasional use of small amounts of lean proteins such as fresh, wild salmon), carefully selected and prepared to suit your particular needs and desires, are ideal foods for your vibrantly alive body. All of these can be eaten either in their natural, uncooked state or after being lightly steamed (avoid fried foods). Complex, processed, fragmented foods can be difficult or impossible for your body to utilize, and eating them is associated with obesity and a host of other problems.

Fat by Design

You may feel that it's too difficult to switch all at once to a new nutritional program. That's a common reaction, but don't think it's because you "lack discipline" or that it's "all in your head." Your body is the result of a countless number of exquisite adaptations that have taken place throughout history. In the scarce environment in which humans lived during most of that time, being able to find and secure the highest-calorie (high-fat, high-sugar) foods was essential for survival. And because these items weren't always available, it was important to be able to put on weight in order to make it through the lean times. It's no surprise that you prefer ice cream to lettuce and pizza to broccoli, and that you go up a dress size if you even look at a cheeseburger.

What's vital for all of us to remember is that in the good old ancestral days, concentrated calories were hard to come by; it was mostly roots and shoots (which is where all the important nutrients come from). In those days, only kings and queens could afford to eat all of the fat-laden animal products and sugary-sweet desserts that you and I can get on any street corner for 99 cents these days. (And because of it, millions of Americans are suffering and dying prematurely from the diseases of kings—heart disease, cancer, diabetes, arthritis, gout, and so on.)

It's not easy to instantly flip the switch on long-established biological adaptations and the eating habits they foster. It's okay to break your ingrained habits gradually, if you wish, switching first to the foods that appeal to you the most and gradually adding the others. In fact, it may take a while for your digestive system to become accustomed to handling the new program. The important thing is that you make changes. Your life depends on it.

Mind Power—Using It to Your Advantage

Like your body, your mind has adapted over the generations of time—with survival as its goal. As you start making positive changes, your mind's adaptations can trip you up if you aren't careful. It always will choose immediate gratification over long-term satisfaction. The mind doesn't care if you achieve your long-term goal for a fit, lean, healthy body; it wants you to feel good right now. It's important to realize that when it comes to pleasure-seeking behavior, what you're thinking isn't necessarily your best friend. You must sometimes override your accustomed habits and "instincts" and make rational decisions about what's actually in your best interest.

In addition to the challenges posed by adaptations, cultural and commercial conditioning contribute to the difficulties you face when you try to resist the temptation to engage in long-established bad habits. Every time you're negatively conditioned, you lose a little of your freedom and your capacity to choose. Begin your new program by becoming aware of what you're eating. Set parameters for yourself—for example, eat only at the dinner table, only at set mealtimes, and/or only when you're hungry. Establishing boundaries helps because they allow you to give your full attention to your food. When your attention is divided, you're more likely to eat compulsively rather than to satiate hunger. Try to minimize the unfocused, "automatic" consumption that frequently occurs in front of the television set and at movie theaters, parties, and sporting events.

To get the maximum benefits of superior nutrition, you need to become mindful of the entire process of eating. Be conscious of the hunger you feel before you begin. How does the food look and smell as you prepare, serve, and consume it? Notice the appearance of the table setting. How does the food taste? Be aware of its texture and monitor how well you chew. Do you make noise when you eat? Be conscious of your breathing and how you feel while you're feeding yourself. After the meal, be aware of, and grateful for, the feelings of lightness and high energy derived from the meal and the ease with which it will be digested. Embracing this attitude toward your meals enables you to appreciate simple, wholesome foods and to feel completely satisfied while eating fewer, higher-nutrient, lower-calorie foods. Enjoying the simplest dishes is one of the keys to unlocking your true health potential.

When you switch from the typical high-calorie, highly processed, "foodless" items that most Americans eat and start choosing whole, natural plant foods, you lose weight naturally. But it's still fun to see excess pounds disappear quickly. To speed up the process and start developing healthier habits at the same time, try this: Stop eating just as you begin to feel full. This technique helps reprogram your subconscious and is a good reminder that you control your habits, not the other way around.

Begin to retrain your senses by eliminating "foods" that injure the body. You wouldn't fill the gas tank of your car with water from a garden hose just because it was easy and inexpensive. You know the car needs a particular type of fuel, lubricant, coolant, and so on. Yet when it comes to yourself (tell the truth), you aren't always so careful. You eat all kinds of things that you know impair the body's smooth functioning. You need to establish new guidelines for eating based on the understanding that the purpose of eating is nourishment. While eating can be very pleasurable, it isn't a form of entertainment designed to appeal to your senses. I've found that meditating for a few minutes before each meal is a powerful tool that fosters intelligent food choices that promote health and harmony.

More than 2,400 years ago, Pythagoras is reported to have said, "Choose what is best; habit will soon render it agreeable and easy." His perspicacious words are just as relevant now as they were in his day, especially when it comes to establishing healthful new food and lifestyle habits. Fortunately, it seems that our taste buds change and adapt when we alter our eating habits, and the whole-grain bread that seemed heavy and grainy a few months ago may be chewy and flavorful this month. Feeling better and looking marvelous will soon compensate for the loss of dubious thrills of the past, such as fried chicken, white bread, ice cream, candy, and potato chips. You'll find yourself looking forward to more healthful pleasures—the taste of ripe papaya; luscious strawberries and blueberries; tangy pineapple; sweet, juicy grapes; a crisp garden salad; brown rice or quinoa with steamed vegetables; and sweet potatoes smothered in steamed or water-sautéed onions, broccoli, and mushrooms.

If you want some healthful, delicious, and easy-to-prepare recipes to add to the ones that appear later in this book, check out my other books: *The Healing Power of NatureFoods, Be Healthy~Stay Balanced,* and *Recipes for Health Bliss: Using NatureFoods to Rejuvenate Your Body & Life* (available from Hay House, June 2009). In all of these works, I bring together the latest and most dramatic findings about what's good and what's deleterious among the things we eat. I show how to make the appropriate food choices to reduce your risks of premature aging, heart disease, common forms of cancer, arthritis, diabetes, depression, and reduced vision and mental function. You'll also learn simple ways to increase energy, boost immunity, beautify skin, improve digestion, and sustain overall great health while losing body fat at the same time.

Change Your Diet, Change Your Life

Let's explore how the life-affirming changes I've been describing benefitted Danielle, one of my clients. She's a great example of how changing your diet and adding more fresh fruits and vegetables and other whole foods can not only assist with weight loss, but also improve every aspect of your life and self-esteem.

Married, with three children (ages 5, 8, and 11), Danielle initially came to me for motivation and help in losing some fat, toning up her body, and increasing her energy. As a first step, I asked her to keep a seven-day food diary and record exactly what and when she ate. Like all of my new clients, she was instructed not to eat differently simply because I'd be looking at the list. I asked her to be honest and write down everything she consumed because there's no other way for me to make a meaningful evaluation.

When I received her food diary, it was quite apparent why she'd gained almost 30 pounds in a year and always felt enervated. Her diet was about 60 percent fat, the carbohydrates she consumed were almost all refined, she usually skipped breakfast because she was too busy getting the children ready for school, and she always ate late at night. Her diary came straight out of my "encyclopedia of deleterious habits." She rarely included raw foods in her diet (or her family's), explaining that they take too long to chew and she didn't have time for that. Danielle also noted that her kids disliked uncooked ingredients, so only on rare occasions did she prepare fruits or vegetables for them.

As I inquired more about her family life, her routines, and so on, I learned that all of her children were on the heavy side, and the oldest girl was being ridiculed in school because of her size. Not surprisingly, Danielle told me that her husband also needed to lose about 40 pounds. His blood pressure, cholesterol, and triglycerides were much too high; and his doctor had suggested that he go on a diet. I told my client that no diet was necessary. Instead, the household needed a health makeover, and I assured her that she'd come to the right person for guidance.

My initial evaluation of what this family ate and how they lived led me to suggest something very out of the ordinary. Knowing that they had a large house with a guest room next to the kitchen, I asked if I could stay with them from Thursday through Saturday night. I wanted to experience their lifestyle as a whole—to see when and what they ate and how they spent their time at home when not eating—in order to coach them in a healthier way of living. Yes, I took most of my own food and simply observed like a butterfly on the wall and took lots of notes. With Danielle's permission, I looked through their pantry and refrigerator and all of their kitchen cupboards. I found hardly any fresh, whole foods.

At mealtimes, everyone added salt to the dishes before even tasting them (using regular table salt is never the ideal thing to do), and their dining table was never without canned sodas or processed fruit juices, butter, sour cream, and mounds of cheese. All five of them ate quickly, without much conversation and without putting the utensils down between bites. To be fair, most of their overeating was unintentional, triggered by the hidden sugar, salt, and oils added to popular foods to stimulate the taste buds.

Danielle and I decided that I should make a clean sweep of her kitchen. The rest of her family went along with this plan, although they were far from enthusiastic. I removed all refined carbohydrates, including pasta, white rice, low-fiber cereals, pancake and cookie mixes, white breads, and bagels. I replaced "foodless" foods with high-fiber breads and whole grains. I also rid their home of margarine, mayonnaise, vegetable shortenings, and oils. Next, I replaced the milk and cheese products with raw nut and seed milks. (It turned out that they all loved the vanilla-flavored almond milk the best after about two weeks of adapting to the new taste.)

I took the entire family to the nearest health-food store, showed them all of the alternatives such as veggie burgers and whole-grain pastas and then, to their amazement, led them into the produce section. They were enthralled by all of the colors and varieties of fruits and vegetables, many of which they'd never seen before. We purchased some of the most familiar—organic apples, oranges, pears, grapes, bananas, and strawberries.

In place of sodas and other canned drinks, I taught them how to make their own juice. The kids loved juicing and actually wanted to take it over as their daily job. Of course, I also encouraged them to start drinking more water. Danielle's husband confessed to me secretly that he couldn't remember ever drinking more than one glass of water a day. When I told him that I drink two to three quarts of purified, alkalinized water every day, he almost collapsed in shock.

It took about one month for the family to adjust their taste buds to the new flavors, textures, and colors of their healthful choices. They basically switched from a white and beige diet to a banquet of rainbow colors. They began eating daily servings of raw foods, with an abundance of fresh fruits and vegetables. When you fill up on these salubrious options, you nourish your body and actually lose much of your desire for sweets and other processed foods.

After three months, I decided to encourage them to consume even more raw foods and showed them many new recipes they could enjoy. They were eager to move in that direction, and after several "non-cooking" lessons, Danielle found it wasn't so hard to prepare more healthful meals. As a result of eating more high-fiber, nutritious ingredients, each family member lost weight, had more energy and more balanced moods, and enjoyed a greater sense of well-being. I encouraged them to be more active, instead of sitting in front of televisions or computers most nights and weekends, and this change resulted in sounder sleep for everyone. Danielle's oldest daughter lost enough weight to join an after-school sports team, which ended the ridicule she'd been enduring and helped her self-esteem soar. It's truly remarkable how a few basic alterations in diet can profoundly affect every area of life.

The change this family found hardest initially, but which ultimately turned out to be the most fun, was my recommendation that they eat only raw food one day each week. I suggested they not pick a weekend day but rather a Tuesday, Wednesday, or Thursday. They selected Thursday, and from morning through evening ate only living foods—lots of fruits and vegetables; salads; and a variety of other fun foods, including nut butters, sprouts, sauces, soups—even cookies and other desserts. The family came to appreciate Danielle's gift for experimenting and creating raw-food meals. A few weeks into their new regimen, they started inviting friends over to sample their delicious "health nut" diet.

As I mentioned above, even though you may not be eager to overhaul your entire approach, at least start by adding more raw, enzyme-rich organic fruits and vegetables to your diet. I recommend the following basic program to almost all of my clients and friends. Each day, make sure that at least 60 percent of the food you put on your plate is uncooked. On Mondays, eat raw items all day until dinner, and on Thursdays, raw foods all day *including* dinner. This simple program will assist you to bring more living foods into your diet by spacing them out over the week. You'll feel lighter and more energetic immediately, simply from eating more raw foods.

Sleepless in America

In addition to restocking Danielle's kitchen with better food choices and urging her family to be more physically active, I also encouraged each of them to make sleep a top priority—a nonnegotiable, nightly habit. Lack of rest undermines your ability to deal with stress and to maintain a healthful weight. One way to tell if you're running short on shut-eye is to see if you wake at a regular time without an alarm. If you require a buzzer to get out of bed in the morning, you're not getting enough sleep.

How much sleep do you really need each day? Adults need 8¼ hours of sleep nightly to maximize their ability to function daily. Adolescents require 9¼ hours; preschoolers have to get 12 hours; toddlers need 13 hours; and babies need 14–18 hours of sleep every day.

Researchers now are discovering that this affects the hormones that regulate satiety, hunger, and how efficiently you burn calories. Put simply, too little sleep makes you hungry, especially for items that are high in calories and low in nutritional value. These include processed junk foods, especially those made with white sugar and flour, and fried foods such as French fries and potato chips. Moreover, lack of sleep also inhibits your body's capacity to rid itself of those extra calories you eat.

Are you interested in slimming down? If so, this may provide some help. Researchers at Columbia University in New York City found that people who slept six hours a night were 23 percent more likely to be obese than those who slept between seven and nine hours. Folks who snoozed for five hours were 50 percent more likely to be obese, and those who slept four hours or less were 73 percent more likely. So if you're eager to drop a few pounds, make getting ample sleep each night a permanent habit in your lifestyle.

In my private practice as well as in my holistic-health seminars around the country, I also recommend increasing quality sleep because it makes for better relationships. If everyone would just make this change and feel more rested, people would be more thoughtful toward each other, and the dynamics of a family would run more smoothly. We'd all be happier and in better moods—adults and children. What a wonderful gift that would be to give to your family, friends, business associates, community, and (if enough people did it) our country. (I'll talk more about the importance of sleep later in the book.)

PART II

✳ ✻ ✳

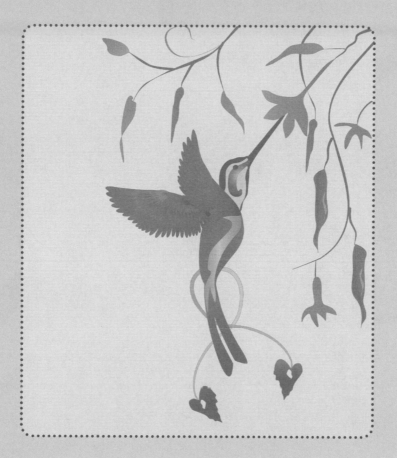

ENTRÉES

50 NATUREFOODS: PART I

"Most people think that you must make enormous changes in your life to be vibrantly healthy. The truth is that it's the simple changes that make the most profound difference."

— SUSAN SMITH JONES

Typically, when people think about advances in health care, they envision new drugs and laser surgeries, high-tech machinery, and innovative surgical techniques. But the most important advances in health care haven't come in the form of medical technology but in scientific knowledge. We now understand that health and vitality (or the absence of them) are rarely caused by chance or heredity and are almost always the result of how we choose to live—including how we eat, sleep, exercise, and manage stress.

For the past 30 years, I've been perusing the scientific literature, conducting my own extensive research, and working with clients around the country and the world on preventing and eliminating disease and creating healthy, balanced lives. In the last decade, studies began to overwhelmingly corroborate my findings—lifestyle changes can prevent and reverse a variety of illnesses and conditions, including heart disease, cancer, all kinds of arthritis, diabetes, obesity, depression, and high blood pressure. Did you know that those last two are the reasons why people visit doctors the most? In 2007, there were a whopping 118 million prescriptions written for antidepressants.

When diet and lifestyle—often the primary causes of poor health—are remedied, the body has a remarkable capacity to begin healing itself. And this happens much more speedily than we'd once thought possible. Conversely, if we ignore the underlying dietary and lifestyle causes of our health woes and try to overcome them with drugs and/or surgery, we run the risk of the same problems recurring and new ones emerging—the so-called side effects. Treating the symptoms of disease with drugs and surgery without eliminating the causes is like mopping up the floor around an overflowing sink without turning off the faucet.

Some of the most dramatic findings published in the most reputable scientific journals show the following:

* Dietary changes can enable diabetic patients to go off their medication.

* Heart disease can be reversed with diet alone.

* Breast cancer is related to levels of female hormones in the blood, which are determined by the food we eat.

* Consuming dairy foods can increase the risk of prostate cancer.

* Antioxidants in colorful fruits and vegetables are linked to better mental performance in old age.

* Kidney stones can be prevented by a healthful diet.

* Type 1 diabetes, one of the most devastating diseases that can overtake a child, is convincingly linked to infant-feeding practices.

These findings demonstrate that a good diet is one of the most powerful weapons we have against disease. An understanding of this scientific evidence is not only important for improving health; it also has profound implications for our entire society. The United States spends far more, per capita, on health care than *any other society in the world,* and yet Americans' health is failing.

Food Choices Are Vitally Important

These findings point to the importance of four things: breakfast, lunch, dinner, and snacks. Irrefutably, food has the potential to harm us and cause us to die younger. As mentioned in the Introduction, it seems that many people (adults and children) are digging their graves with their forks and knives. And sadly, it's now taking a toll on our younger generation. Here are some raw facts about our youth and the noxious obesity epidemic sweeping this country:

❋ Many youngsters today won't live as long as their parents— for the first time in history.

❋ 80 percent of type 2 diabetes cases are related to obesity.

❋ 70 percent of heart disease cases are related to obesity.

❋ One in four obese children contemplates suicide.

❋ More American kids were killed by obesity-related illnesses than gun violence in 2006.

We've got to change things. One of the reasons I wrote my children's nutrition book *Vegetable Soup/The Fruit Bowl* (co-authored with Dianne Warren) was to help reverse the above statistics and help children start off in a positive direction. This book is the ideal way to lay the groundwork for lifelong healthful eating habits. Every child deserves this unique volume. What better gift can you give them as they grow than vitality and radiant health? (For more information on this book or to order it, please visit my Website: **www.SusanSmithJones.com**.)

A Plant-Based Diet Is Best

More scientific evidence than ever points to the fact that switching from a high-fat diet rich in animal-protein foods and simple carbohydrates (such as sugar and white-flour products) to a colorful whole-foods (mostly plant-based) diet high in complex carbohydrates provides double benefits. *You significantly reduce your intake of disease-promoting substances—such as cholesterol, saturated and trans fats, and oxidants—and increase your intake of protective food substances.*

In foods, there are at least 1,000 substances—including bioflavonoids, isoflavones, carotenoids, phytochemicals, lycopene, and genistein—that have anticancer, anti–heart disease, and antiaging properties. Where are these found? With very few exceptions, they're all in the plant-based foods—in fruits, vegetables, grains, beans, nuts, and seeds.

If you want to eat bacon and eggs with white-bread toast and margarine for breakfast, washed down with a few cups of coffee, that's your prerogative. The problem is that you'll end up taking cholesterol and blood-pressure medication and antacids, hoping against the odds that they'll prolong your debilitated life. But if you truly want to take charge of your health, read every page of this book carefully (as well as *The Healing Power of NatureFoods*). If you heed the advice I offer, you'll thank yourself every day for the rest of your life.

Clearly, Western medicine doesn't have the answers to most chronic health problems, as witnessed by the many billions of dollars spent each year to try to find cures for conditions such as heart disease, cancers, obesity, and diabetes. That is why I believe that people are now ready to go back to basics and let nature do what it does best—*keep us healthy.*

Nature's Best Foods

As you peruse the upcoming 50 salubrious NatureFoods, keep in mind the following thought: In nature, you won't find white-bread trees, ice-cream bushes, potato-chip vines, or French-fry plants. The best things to eat are the naturally colorful and fiber-rich plant foods I'm about to describe. The more of these you include in your meal, the more healthful nutrients you'll get. Those will boost immunity, protect your body from disease, accelerate fat loss, and promote radiant health and vibrancy.

Choose to eat foods in a rainbow of colors, as close to the way nature made them as possible. And keep in mind that raw items (enzyme- and nutrient-rich, live-food cuisine) play an important role in an optimal diet. Here's a good way to think about it: *Produce is the most important health care your money can buy.*

As with *The Healing Power of NatureFoods,* my goal is to inspire you to transform your diet and zest for life by describing and emphasizing the very best benefits of the very best foods. However, I don't want to give the impression that you must precisely micromanage every meal, depending on how you're feeling that day, week, month, or year. Remember, while I'm singing the praises of these best-of-the-best choices and describing their extraordinary health benefits, keep in mind that *all fresh fruits, vegetables, legumes, raw nuts and seeds, and whole grains bring tremendous benefits.* The unsurpassed nutrients and other qualities I describe for individual foods also can be found in varying degrees in *all* of the NatureFoods that I recommend for a complete, overall healthful diet.

Don't limit yourself to just those fruits and vegetables that you can find anywhere—apples, bananas, oranges, grapes, lettuce, tomatoes, peas, and carrots.

By adding a wide variety of fruits and vegetables to your diet, you expand your body's intake of flavonoids, phytonutrients, vitamins, minerals, enzymes, and other key nutrients. A combination of these may have a greater protective benefit than each one on its own.

Rated for Health

As I describe the NatureFoods in this book, I sometimes refer to a food's ORAC score. The acronym ORAC stands for "Oxygen Radical Absorbance Capacity"; this is a test that measures how effectively the antioxidants found in foods work in your system to fight against oxidative stress. Foods with high ORAC scores are wonderful additions to a healthful diet. (Researchers suggest that we shoot for an overall daily total of about 3,500 units.) Another term I frequently refer to is RDA, the acronym for "Recommended Daily Allowance," which is the amount of each of the various nutrients you need to ingest each day as determined by the U.S. Department of Agriculture (USDA).

I've organized my list of foods in alphabetical order so that after you've read everything, it will be easy to look back and find your favorites. Sound simple enough? Okay, let's get started.

Açai Berries

Pronounced *ah SIGH-ee*, this little purple fruit (less than an inch in diameter) grows wild in strings on the açai palm tree in the lush rain forests of South America. A nutritional powerhouse of health and healing, the açai berry has been around for thousands of years, and local tribes have used it as a cure for various ailments, claiming that it possesses a wealth of salubrious properties. Now modern science has discovered the myriad benefits of this exotic fruit.

Açai berries contain amino acids and vital trace elements important for muscle contraction and regeneration. They also have ample dietary fiber (excellent for digestive tract health) and high levels of calcium, vitamins A and E, and phosphorus. They're an excellent source of antioxidants, boasting high concentrations of polyphenols, including especially potent anthocyanins. The berries are a great source of essential fatty acids (omega-3 and omega-6) plus oleic acid (omega-9), which are good for lowering low-density lipoprotein (LDL) levels, and they're rich in phytosterols (compounds of plant cell membranes) that help reduce blood pressure.

The tribes of the Amazon knew of these healthful properties and used the açai to fight disease, strengthen immune function, combat infection, protect the heart, and enhance overall health and healing. This berry has great potential as a super-antioxidant supplement, which is why I've selected it as one of my 50 NatureFoods.

The USDA reports: "Young and middle-aged people may be able to reduce the risk of the diseases of aging (including senility) simply by adding high-ORAC foods to their diets." Fruits high in antioxidants include açai berries, cranberries, pomegranates, blueberries, peaches, camu camu, kiwis, grapes, and prunes. The higher a food's ORAC score, the better it is in fighting damage from oxidative stress and helping your body combat degenerative diseases such as cancer, memory loss, and heart disease.

The açai berries score extremely well on the ORAC test. Based on USDA data, *the açai berry is 500–1,000 percent higher in antioxidant activity than any other fruit or vegetable known to humankind!* Doctors recommend 3,000–5,000 ORAC units per day in your diet. Per gram, the ORAC scores for some sample foods are: wild blueberries 260, red raspberries 210, spinach 150, broccoli 130, cherries 100, green beans 70, and carrots 50. Açai comes in at a whopping 1,026.

The benefits of these berries are now available in teas and juices. I purchase a variety of açai drinks at natural-food stores and general supermarkets. They're either plain or blended with the juices of other fruits such as blueberry, raspberry, mango, pomegranate, or passion fruit.

In addition, the açai berry may help . . .

* Enhance muscle contractions and muscle regeneration
* Protect blood vessels
* Prevent osteoporosis
* Reduce bad cholesterol
* Improve the function of immune cells
* Aid in weight control
* Improve glucose and lipid levels
* Heal ulcers
* Reduce arthritis pain
* Aid vision

* Improve mental clarity
* Act as an antimutogenic
* Thwart viruses, bacterial infections, and funguses
* Lower blood pressure
* Prevent free-radical damage to the immune system
* Promote better sleep

If you haven't yet experienced this amazing berry, you're in for a real treat. I always have fresh açai tea ready to enjoy and also a few bottles of açai juice chilling in my refrigerator. Whether I drink it plain or in combination with other juices, or use it as a base for my smoothies or fruit sauces, it's one of my favorite antioxidant-rich berry drinks.

Aloe Vera

This ancient, unassuming, cactus-type member of the lily family is easily overlooked. Nevertheless, it's one of the most outstanding medicinal plants in history. It's botanical name is *Aloe barbadensis. Aloe* comes from the Arabic word for "bitter, clear, shining substance," while *vera* is a Latin word meaning "true." A perennial succulent, it has stiff, lance-shaped, spiked leaves that are filled with a clear, gel-like, mucilaginous substance.

References to research on the healing effects of aloe vera have appeared in many authoritative medical publications, such as the *Journal of Pharmaceutical Sciences, Oral Surgery, Cancer, Industrial Medicine and Surgery,* and the *International Journal of Dermatology.* These studies address aloe's use in a broad range of conditions, including acne, leg ulcers, digestive disorders, radiation burns, and dental surgery.

Skin healing often requires increased blood flow to the injured area, and aloe vera dilates capillaries, which increases circulation and speeds recovery. The plant is an especially effective treatment in cases of frostbite. It also helps heal all sores, from canker sores to bed sores, as well as burns, abrasions, herpes lesions, hives, insect bites and stings, scalp itchiness, psoriasis, and sunburn pain. (*Trop Med Int. Health* 1(4):505–509, 1996 and *J. Med. Assoc. Thai.* 78(8):403–409, 1995)

Because of its amazing anti-inflammatory action in the digestive system, aloe also has been found to be effective in the treatment of heartburn, peptic ulcers, and constipation; and it has potential as a remedy for Crohn's disease and ulcerative colitis.

After decades of laboratory analysis, scientists still can only partially explain aloe vera's incredible nontoxic potency. The plant appears to increase the rate of healing in the intercellular matrix, thus strengthening new tissue as it forms. Aloe contains gamma linoleic acid, which decreases inflammation, and it's loaded with a storehouse of other nutrients—including vitamins B_1, B_2, B_3, B_6, C, and choline—plus the minerals calcium, chlorine, copper, germanium, iron, magnesium lactate, manganese, potassium, silicon, sodium, and sulfur. But its uniqueness lies in its wealth of phytochemicals (such as the organic acids chrysophanic, salicylic, succinic, and uric), polysaccharides (such as acemannan and enzymes such as glutathione peroxidase), and various resins.

Although the use of aloe gel on the skin is well known, little attention has been given to the amazing effects of drinking properly prepared aloe-vera juice. In fact, the plant has an amazing number of healthful effects when ingested orally. Research has shown that it stimulates the fibroblasts to produce new tissue, which means that collagen, proteoglycans, and other cofactors also create new tissue.

Additionally, aloe's anti-inflammatory and analgesic properties aid in soothing irritated tissues and promoting healthy linings and repair. These regenerative qualities help rebuild the stomach, the small and large intestines, and the colon.

Aloe polysaccharides may also have properties that enhance the gastrointestinal system. These substances improve the activity of immune cells, improving their ability to kill bacteria and viruses and cleanse and eliminate waste and toxic buildup.

For the optimal supply of this NatureFood, keep a decorative aloe plant in your home, as I always do. No green thumb required, as it's attractive and easy to maintain. For external use, snip a piece of leaf, split it open, and dab the gel on burns, irritated skin, or wounds. For a beverage, scrape off two tablespoons of gel from a split leaf, stir into a glass of water or juice, and drink. I often include fresh aloe-vera gel in my morning or afternoon smoothie—just blend it with your preferred fresh fruits and other ingredients. I also throw some of the snipped-off green leaf into my juicer along with my favorite fruits.

If you're purchasing aloe vera, keep this in mind: Look for a product that's *unrefined* or unfiltered; the plant must be purified without *any* heat whatsoever. Unfortunately, cold-processed aloe vera doesn't mean that it's "raw" (uncooked) since it's actually "flash heated," according to Jeri L. Heyman, a renowned aloe researcher. Finding a completely raw product is the key. If it's heated at all, it isn't going to be as potent or effective as the raw substance. My favorite juice and skin gel is made by Herbal Force; to order, visit: **www.herbalanswers.com** or call (888) 256-3367.

Apricots

To those who have meandered amid apricot trees bearing ripe fruit, it makes perfect sense that apricot nectar was called the "fruit of the gods." Though my dictionary doesn't associate this NatureFood with nectar, common usage does, and it's a link that I've never doubted. Apricot's malic- and citric-acid content give a lemony bite to this otherwise sweet, buttery fruit, a plum relative that originated in Asia. Today, California produces 90 percent of the domestic apricot crop.

The fruit's unique mix of healing compounds makes it a powerful ally in protecting the eyes and preventing heart disease. It's rich in beta-carotene and lycopene, compounds that have been shown in studies to fight the process by which the dangerous low-density lipoprotein (LDL) form of cholesterol turns rancid in the bloodstream. This is important because when LDL goes bad, it's more likely to stick to artery walls. "Lycopene is currently considered one of the strongest antioxidants we know about," says Frederick Khachik, Ph.D., research chemist at the USDA Food Composition Laboratory in Beltsville, Maryland.

A 13-year study found that those with the highest intakes of carotenoids had a one-third lower risk of heart disease than those with the lowest intakes. In an eight-year study of 90,000 nurses, those with the diets richest in carotenoids had a 25 percent lower risk. Other compounds in this velvety fruit have been found to fight infections and blindness. A study of more than 50,000 nurses found that women who got the most vitamin A in their diets reduced their risk of getting cataracts by more than one-third. Three apricots provide 2,769 IU of vitamin A, 55 percent of the RDA.

In addition to being a good source of vitamin C, apricots are rich in beta-carotene, with three apricots containing 2 mg, about 30 percent of the RDA. Much of the vitamin C is lost, however, when they're canned or dried in high heat. In all forms, apricots are high in iron and potassium, a mineral essential for proper nerve and muscle function that also helps maintain normal blood pressure and balance of body fluids.

I purchase pounds of organic apricots, when they're in season, and dry them in my dehydrator (below 110 degrees to retain nutrients and enzymes) to enjoy year-round. The best ones available already dried come from Turkey. Keep a container of these delights in your desk drawer for mid-afternoon munchies. Avoid apricots that are treated with sulfur dioxide. This sulfite treatment may trigger an asthma attack or allergic reaction in susceptible people. In other words, unless they're labeled as sulfite free, anyone with asthma should avoid them.

Here are a couple of storage tips. It's important to keep apricots cool to prevent them from getting overripe. Unless you're going to eat them within a day or two, it's best to store them in the fruit bin in the refrigerator, where they'll keep for about a week. Because they readily pick up flavors from other fruits they're stored with (and even from refrigerator smells), it's a good idea to keep them in a paper or plastic bag.

Artichokes

"Back in 1948, Marilyn Monroe's first claim to fame was being crowned California's Artichoke Queen. Today, artichokes need little endorsement," writes Rebecca Wood in *The New Whole Food Encyclopedia*. Served either hot or cold, they're both a delicacy and a low-calorie, nutritious vegetable. One medium artichoke has only 65 calories, but it provides 28 percent of the RDA of folate, 16 percent of the RDA of vitamin C, 10 percent of the RDA of potassium, and about three grams of fiber. Artichokes also contain *cynarin,* an organic acid that stimulates the sweetness receptors in the taste buds of some people, causing the foods eaten afterward to taste sweeter.

A member of the sunflower—or composite—plant family, artichokes provide a variety of heart-healthy phytochemicals. In a recent German study, 143 patients with high cholesterol were given either 1,800 milligrams of dry artichoke extract or a placebo every day for six weeks. At the end, those taking the extract had reduced their total cholesterol by 18 percent on average and had lowered their "bad" cholesterol by 23 percent, resulting in a better overall ratio of HDL to LDL—nearly as great an improvement as with medication. At least part of the effect was likely due to cynarin, which increases the liver's production of bile. That substance, in turn, helps the body remove cholesterol.

In a study at the University Hospitals of Cleveland and Case Western Reserve University School of Medicine, also in Cleveland, researchers found that an ointment made with *silymarin,* a compound (consisting of a group of flavonoids) found in artichoke hearts, was able to prevent skin cancer in mice. "Silymarin works because it is a powerful antioxidant," explains researcher Hasan Mukhtar, Ph.D., professor of dermatology and environmental health sciences at Case Western Reserve University School of Medicine. "It's such an effective antioxidant that silymarin extract is even used medicinally against liver disease in Europe."

Antioxidants help prevent cancer in the body by mopping up harmful, cell-damaging molecules known as free radicals before they damage DNA and pave the way for tumors to develop. You can't stop free radicals from forming, but artichokes can block their effects. And unless you dine on milk thistle, which few people do, artichokes are likely to be the only place that you'll find silymarin in your diet.

In another study, this one at the AMC Cancer Research Center in Denver, silymarin was used topically on skin cancers in mice. The results were startling. According to cancer biologist Rajesh Agarwal, "It reduced the number of mice who developed cancers by 75 percent." Those that did develop tumors had 92 percent fewer cancers, and the tumor size was 97 percent smaller. "In cancer research, that's as good as it gets," he says. (He has since begun giving the animals silymarin orally to see if it can prevent prostate tumors, too.)

With all of this good news about artichokes and skin health, you also may want to try one of my favorite facial masks by Reviva called the Optimum Antioxidant Facial Mask with Artichoke. It's a "super cocktail" for your skin. I refer to it as a "booster shot" for the skin's immune system; it's a defense against future damage from UV rays, pollution, stress, and poor diet. I've used this product once a week for years and recommend it to all of my friends and clients. It makes my skin healthy and youthful-looking. You can find this superlative facial mask in your health-food store. To order it directly from the company, visit: **www.revivalabs.com** or call: (800) 257-7774.

Unfortunately, you won't get enough silymarin from artichokes to guarantee a cancer-free existence, but one of these vegetables every now and then clearly can't hurt. They can be one more weapon in your disease-fighting arsenal.

Simmer artichokes for about 50 minutes, or pressure-cook them for only 15 minutes. Because they discolor easily, keep them covered in acidulated water (water plus a little lemon juice or vinegar). Exposure to air can cause them to turn a grayish color. Baby artichokes may be trimmed, then halved or quartered, and sautéed or baked. If you plant this vegetable in your garden, plan for enough for eating and then some extra for their mature blossoms. Dried or fresh, artichoke flowers make a stunning floral display. Whether for consumption or to increase the resplendence of your garden, this vegetable deserves center stage.

Arugula

Going by the names of rocket, roquette, and rugola, the leafy green arugula has a distinct, peppery bite and resembles dandelion greens. It used to be sold only in Italian markets, but is now widely available year-round. One of my all-time favorite salad ingredients, the younger (and smaller) arugula has a less pungent bite. Look for emerald-green leaves two to four inches in length; avoid if the leaves are yellowing or limp. You usually can find it sold in bunches with the roots still attached or already washed and in bags, ready to toss into a salad and enjoy. Because arugula is highly perishable, immediately wrap the roots in a damp paper towel as soon as you get home from the store. Enclose in a plastic bag or other container and refrigerate for no more than three days.

To prepare, wash thoroughly by chopping off the roots and any thick stems and swishing the leaves up and down in a sink full of cold water. Let stand for a minute or so. Swirl the leaves around again, wait another minute, and then remove.

In the ancient world, arugula was considered to possess aphrodisiac properties; it was sown around the bases of statues consecrated to Priapus and believed to restore vigor to the genitalia. The early Christian church knew of its supposed erotic properties and frowned upon its use and cultivation. Today, the oil extracted from its seeds is still used in Europe as an aphrodisiac.

Arugula is rich in beta-carotene and higher in vitamin C than many other leafy greens. It also provides vitamin A, niacin, iron, and phosphorus and is good for normalizing body acid with its high alkalinity. Additionally, because one of its key minerals is sulfur, it helps prevent ridges in your nails. It's versatile, delicious, and a great choice to add pizzazz to any meal.

Barley Grass

Cereal grasses such as barley, wheat, rye, and oats have long been cultivated for their energy-dense grain, but the most nutritious part of these plants resides in their young, green blades of grass. Although stored grain retains its nutrient value for long periods, the leaves begin to lose their nutrition shortly after being cut. Fortunately, modern-day processing techniques now exist to capture and stabilize the abundant nutrients in freshly harvested grass, making its everyday use practical.

For optimal health, we need to consume both macronutrients (proteins, fats, and carbohydrates) and micronutrients (including vitamins, minerals, amino acids, active enzymes, carotenoids, bioflavonoids, chlorophyll, and other phytochemicals). Of the green cereal grasses, barley grass is especially rich in micronutrients, and a comparative analysis found that it contained the most balanced nutritional profile out of 150 different green plants. It provides essential nutrients necessary for cellular function and contains phytochemicals that promote growth and development, enhance metabolism, control inflammation, protect against free radicals and toxins, enhance the immune system, and may increase longevity.

And speaking of longevity, as we age, both immune function and growth-hormone levels decline, thereby reducing the body's ability to protect and repair itself. Dr. Allan L. Goldstein, at George Washington School of Medicine, found that barley-grass juice contains a special type of vitamin E (vitamin E succinate) that increases production of growth hormone and may enhance the immune system by increasing white-blood-cell formation.

Other new research found that young barley-grass extracts effectively degraded a variety of organophosphorus pesticides, including malathion, chlorpyrifos, guthion, diazinon, methidathion, and parathion. Incubation of the individual pesticides with a 3 percent solution of barley-grass juice for several hours resulted in the complete degradation of both malathion and chlorpyrifos along with a significant breakdown of parathion by 75 percent, diazinon by 54 percent, guthion by 41 percent, and methidathion by 23 percent. It also was confirmed that barley-grass juice's ability to break down malathion is lost when the grass is heated to 120° C, most likely due to destruction of enzyme activity by heat.

Adding barley-grass juice powder (processed at low temperatures so it's still considered raw) to your diet is a convenient and effective way to ensure that you reap the benefits of nature's green bounty, which provides those phytonutrients and phytochemicals necessary for maintaining optimal health. I mix barley powder into my smoothies, juices, teas, soups, and dips and stir it into a large glass of purified water. It's also the perfect, versatile supplement to take with you (in a plastic storage bag) on trips.

For a tasty and colorful barley boost to my diet, I use BarleyMax several times weekly in a variety of recipes, including juices. This concentrated barley-juice powder is convenient to use and absolutely delicious. It boasts the following properties: It's made from certified organic barley grass; it's made by a low-temperature drying process that retains critical heat-sensitive nutrients and living enzymes; it has no sweeteners or artificial ingredients; and it mixes easily with water to make a rich, nutritious juice. Offered exclusively through Hallelujah Acres (**www.hacres.com**), it's created through a proprietary dehydration process that's capable of transforming juice to a powder with minimal degradation of color, flavor, aroma, enzymes, and nutrients. (I also recommend their BeetMax and CarrotJuiceMax powders. Mixing the three together makes a delicious, quick, and rejuvenating drink.)

Berries

The cheery bright red of cranberries and strawberries and the rich dark blue of blackberries and blueberries are not only beautiful to behold, but these and other luscious hues also benefit human beings with their healthful properties. One of the most underrated of all fruit categories, berries (especially if they're organically grown) benefit all body systems and people of all ages. Raspberries and strawberries are among the fruits highest in pesticides if not grown organically, while blueberries are among the lowest.

If you take a look at the ORAC scores for a variety of different fruits, you'll see that berries consistently take the prize for their richness. Here's a sampling of ORAC scores for 3½ ounces of antioxidant-rich fruits:

kiwi 602	raspberries 1,220
cherries 670	strawberries 1,540
grapes 739	cranberries 1,750
oranges 750	blackberries 2,036
avocado 782	blueberries 2,400
plums 949	raisins 2,830
	prunes 5,770

In a study at The Ohio State University, scientists found that berries reduced the risk of malignant colon tumors by 80 percent. The substances believed to bring about this anticancer effect are antioxidants called anthocyanins, the pigments that give these berries their dark color. "We were surprised by how much difference there was between the antioxidant activity of the raspberries versus other fruits," says Gary Stoner, Ph.D., co-author of the study and professor of public health at Ohio State (*Nutr Can* 4/02). In Dr. Stoner's study, the more berries the animals ate, the less cancer they developed. Tests performed by the researchers suggested that free radicals, caustic molecules whose action can lead to cancer and other health problems, were absorbed by the berries' antioxidants.

Researchers are also excited about a class of health-boosting chemicals called phenols. Blackberries contain them, but the queen of this category may be the cranberry. An antioxidant comparison of some of the most common fruits found that cranberries contain the most of this type of antioxidant, which is thought to reduce the risk of cancer, stroke, and heart disease (*J Agri Food Chem* 11/19/01). One investigation found that a daily glass of this tart beverage can raise "good" HDL cholesterol by about 10 percent, which translates to about a 40 percent reduction in heart disease risk. As most people know, cranberries also have been long used for urinary-tract health.

Because blueberries and blackberries are two of my favorite fruits, I include them in smoothies and fruit salads, blend them into purées, and simply eat them out of hand. Known as an excellent laxative, blood cleanser, and antioxidant, they're the only food that has been shown to prevent *and to reverse* abnormal physical and mental decline.

— **Blueberries:** Native to North America, blueberries have been part of the human diet for more than 13,000 years and rank among the best foods you can eat. I recommend having them (either fresh or frozen) several times a week. When I can't get them fresh, I always have frozen organic blueberries on hand and use them when making smoothies.

They're good for dieters, too. One cup of blueberries contains only 80 calories, and a whole pint gives you just 180 calories. Like all foods, the calories in these berries come from their *macro*nutrients—56 grams of carbohydrate, 1.5 grams of fat, and 2.7 grams of protein. But it's blueberries' *micro*nutrient content that packs the most impressive wallop.

Referred to as the "brain berry," these little wonders are packed with red pigments (the anthocyanins I mentioned previously) that have been linked to the prevention—and even reversal—of age-related mental decline and anticancer effects. They're one of the most potent antidotes to oxidative stress, a process that ages you. The flavonoids in blueberries—catechin, epicatechin, myricetin, quercetin, and kaempferol—are more than a mouthful of strangely spelled words; they're extremely valuable for superior health. Blueberries are to fruit what broccoli is to vegetables. Is there any higher praise?

— **Blackberries:** Part of the year, I live in Oregon. One of my favorite times to be there is in the summer when the antioxidant-rich fruit, the bodacious blackberry, is ready to pick fresh and enjoy. At the top of Oregon's noxious weed list, it's also ranked among the state's most promising farm crops. A very recent study has found the berries' antioxidant properties to be unmatched, while additional current research has identified a blackberry extract that reduces cancerous tumors in animals. Scientists keep finding more ways this fruit promotes health. *Even a half cup a day of the black fruits (such as blackberries, black raspberries, boysenberries, and loganberries) is significant for fighting many different diseases.* The blueberry story started the berry phenomenon. Now, blackberries are getting a chance to be part of the action—and glorified, as they should be.

The baby boomers want to live forever. We're starting to look at diet as a preventive measure for everything that's going on. Finally! Keep company with berries.

Burdock Root

Also known as gobo root and burr, among other names, burdock root is popular in Japan and can be found in Asian groceries and many health-food stores. Inside its scruffy exterior is a grayish white flesh with a sweet, earthy flavor and a crisp, tender texture. It grows wild in North America; the plant can be recognized by its very large leaves and spiny burrs (the "cockleburs") that stick to your clothes when you walk through a meadow.

Choose firm burdock roots. If the outside is dirty or muddy, don't let that be a deterrent to buying this vegetable; just wash the root well. If the skin is thin, you need not peel it. Cut the vegetable into chunks, slices, or shreds with a sharp, heavy knife. It can be juiced, cooked, or added to salads and other dishes. Tender young burdock leaves have a slightly bitter flavor but are wonderful in salads; and the stems of older plants can be peeled, steamed, and served like asparagus.

Don't cook this food in an aluminum or iron pot, because it can react with the metal to discolor both pot and plant.

The health benefits of the burdock root make it a venerable NatureFood. It has large concentrations of vitamins and minerals, especially iron, and is actually higher in minerals than beets, carrots, potatoes, or turnips. It has more protein, calcium, and phosphorus than carrots and is an excellent source of potassium. Depending on the variety, burdock is 27–45 percent inulin, a form of starch that's easily digested (good for diabetics) and the source of most of its curative powers.

Burdock is one of the great alternative herbs, restoring the body to normal health by cleansing and purifying the blood, supporting digestion and the elimination of toxins, and helping restore normal body functions. In both European and Asian natural-healing centers, burdock formulas are recommended as an anticarcinogen. German researchers confirmed antitumor activity in all parts of burdock as long ago as 1964. It's also given as a treatment for arthritis, as a liver detoxifier, and for general kidney support.

Burdock tea helps heal all kinds of skin diseases, boils, and carbuncles. It also has a stimulating effect on the metabolism and gently but persistently activates and tones all of the organs of elimination, thus inducing a process of inner cleansing. To add to this partial list of contributors to burdock's venerable status, the Chinese also consider the plant to be a strengthening aphrodisiac.

Burdock is definitely a NatureFood that you want to make part of your regular dict so that you can reap all of its benefits.

Cabbage

Like other members of the cruciferous vegetable family, cabbage is one of the most beneficial foods we have. Hundreds of varieties are grown throughout the world, but in American markets you'll find four basic kinds: green, red (or purple), savoy, and various types of Chinese cabbage.

Ancient Roman healers thought that they could cure breast cancer by rubbing on pastes made from cabbage. A few years ago, modern scientists would have dismissed that practice as folklore. Now, they're not so sure.

"Studies have shown that if you make cabbage into a paste and rub it on the backs of laboratory animals, you can prevent tumors from developing," says Jon Michnovicz, M.D., Ph.D., president of the Foundation for Preventive Oncology in New York City. Of course, the best way to absorb the healing properties of cabbage is simply to eat it. The plant not only fights off a variety of cancers (breast, prostate, and colon) but also contains a wealth of nutrients that can ward off heart disease, digestive problems, and other conditions.

There are two compounds in particular that scientists believe make cabbage a potent cancer-fighting food. The first of these, indole-3-carbinol or I3C, is especially effective against breast cancer, research shows. The compound acts as an antiestrogen, meaning that it sweeps up harmful estrogens that have been linked to the disease. Half a head of cabbage each day may be enough to help prevent certain forms of cancer, especially breast. Researchers believe that indoles—nitrogen compounds in this NatureFood and other cruciferous vegetables—play an important protective role. For even more protection, try replacing your usual cabbage with bok choy, or Chinese cabbage, which comes as a celery-like stalk of white leaves. Research has found that a substance in this plant called *brassinin* may help prevent breast tumors.

Cabbage contains another compound, sulforaphane, which has been shown to block cancer by stepping up the production of tumor-preventing enzymes in the body. This makes the plant a particularly prized fighter in the battle against colon cancer, adds Dr. Michnovicz, because it stimulates levels of an enzyme called glutathione in the colon, which researchers believe sweeps toxins out of the body before they have a chance to damage the delicate cells lining the intestinal wall.

Consuming any kind of cabbage on a regular basis probably will lower your risk for cancer. To get the best possible protection, researchers recommend savoy cabbage. It contains not only I3C and sulforaphane but also four other tongue-twisting phytonutrients—beta-sitosterol, pheophytin-a, nonacosane, and nonacosanone—that studies show are powerful contenders against potential cancer-causing agents. Bok choy is healthful, too, and is very high in calcium.

Another remarkable attribute of cabbage is its power to cure ulcers. One study proved that a seven-day regimen of cabbage juice—one quart per day—works wonders on peptic ulcers. Of the 65 patients who participated in the study, 63 were cured! Even the best of today's pharmaceutical remedies can't claim such success. Drinking freshly made cabbage juice works wonders with duodenal, jejunal, and gastric ulcers.

High levels of the minerals potassium, iron, calcium, sulfur, phosphorus, and iodine are found in cabbage, plus the vitamins A, B_1, B_2, B_6, C, E, K, and folic acid. To best take advantage of these wonderful nutrients, try to eat the food raw. If that's too hard for you to digest, the next best way to get your cabbage is to juice it. Also try cabbage sprouts. They're delicate and easier to digest, and they contain higher levels of nutrients. You can put them in the juicer, too.

So the next time you go grocery shopping, fill your cart with one of your body's best friends. Cabbage is versatile, inexpensive, readily available, and easy to prepare. A head will keep for up to ten days in the crisper drawer, making it easy to eat a little bit each day without worrying about it spoiling. Keep your refrigerator well stocked with this illustrious vegetable.

Cauliflower

Mark Twain once called cauliflower "nothing but cabbage with a college education." What he didn't know is that the vegetable can be a valuable asset in the quest for vibrant health. Like other members of the cruciferous family, it's loaded with nutrients that seem to wage war against a host of diseases, including cancer. It's also an excellent source of vitamins and minerals that are essential for keeping the immune system strong.

Although its darker-colored sister, broccoli, has gotten most of the attention for its healing potential, cauliflower also is generously endowed with cancer-preventing powers. In fact, this filling, high-fiber, low-calorie vegetable (only 25 calories in a cup of florets) is one of the most powerful healing foods you can eat. That same one-cup portion has more than 100 percent of the RDA of vitamin C, a third of the RDA for folate (the plant source of folic acid), and reasonable amounts of potassium and vitamin B_6. It also contains bioflavonoids and other chemicals that protect against cancer.

Researchers have found two potent munitions in cauliflower's cancer-fighting arsenal: the phytonutrients sulforaphane and indole-3-carbinol, or I3C. These compounds, which are found in all cruciferous vegetables, may be the reason why research consistently shows that people who make a habit of crunching crucifers are less likely to get cancer.

In one study, scientists at Johns Hopkins University in Baltimore exposed 145 laboratory animals to high doses of an extremely powerful cancer-causing agent. Of those, 120 were given high levels of protective sulforaphane. After 50 days, 68 percent of the unprotected animals had breast tumors, compared with only 26 percent of those that received the sulforaphane. This substance works by stepping up the production of enzymes in your body that sweep toxins out the door before they can damage your body's cells, making them cancerous.

To make sure cauliflower's cancer-fighting indoles remain intact, keep it out of the heat. Your best bet is either eating it raw or cooking it quickly in a steamer, wok, or microwave. Boiling is the worst way to prepare this crucifer. Submerging it in the hot, roily water will cause it to lose about half of its valuable indoles. I sometimes include cauliflower as one of the key ingredients in my fresh vegetable juices.

Cherimoya

Pronounced *cheh-ree-MOY-a*, the cherimoya is part of a family of flowering plants called the *Annonaceae,* also known by the general name of custard apple. These flowering plants produce some of the world's most delicious fruit. Of these, the cherimoya is the most well-known, most commercially available, and most highly prized premium fruit. Mark Twain called it "the most delicious fruit known to man."

The Incan word *cherimoya* means "cold seeds." This luscious NATUREFOOD has also been referred to as "the fruit of the Incas," "the pearl of the Andes," and "the queen of subtropical fruits." According to Latin American lore, the heart-shaped cherimoya is thought of as conducive to romance, best shared with a loved one. The ancient Incas used it as an aphrodisiac and to help improve fertility.

It's believed that the plant originated in the Andean valleys of Peru and Ecuador. It has been grown for centuries throughout the South American tropical highlands and temperate areas. Columbus's explorers discovered it in the Caribbean, and it was one of the first American fruits transported back to Spain.

These richly sweet, semitropical fruits typically have fragrant, custardy, ivory pulp, although the flesh of the *selma* cherimoya variety is pink. Annonaceae flesh is higher in sugar and protein than most other fruits, and little compares to the wonderful taste of a ripe cherimoya. It's slightly acidulous with its lemony tang and exotic, musky overtones; it's also known for its silky, sensuous, melting texture. I think it has a decidedly tropical taste—part mango, part pineapple, part banana.

When the skin becomes slightly soft and the fruit emanates a perfume-like fragrance, it's ripe. Slice it in wedges or halves, and scoop out the flesh with a spoon. When frozen and run through a food processor or Champion juicer, it makes the ultimate fruit sorbet. I also use this fruit in salads, sauces, drinks, smoothies, and desserts and as an ice cream.

Scattered at random throughout the cherimoya are quite a few black seeds, similar to those found in watermelons, which are inedible. I just spit out the seeds as I dig my spoon into the flesh. Each bite will provide you with a variety of nutrients, including calcium, phosphorus, vitamin C, some of the B vitamins, beta-carotene, and fiber.

Cherimoyas are mostly available in the winter and early spring. They may vary in size from half a pound to two pounds; the size doesn't alter the flavor. Because they're harvested while still hard, let them ripen at home. Avoid purchasing ones that are brown or bruised. To increase sweetness, allow cherimoyas to ripen at room temperature just until they begin to brown, but before they become overly soft. Once ripe, they may be refrigerated for up to five days. (Don't refrigerate them before they soften.) Handle them gently, as the skins aren't as tough as they appear to be, and savor every bite.

If you've never tried a cherimoya, treat yourself to this wonderful fruit. Here are a couple of simple ways to use them: Blend together one avocado and two cherimoyas; remove the pit, seeds, and skins first, of course. This combination will dazzle your taste buds. You can also combine two cups of baby spinach, one avocado, and one cherimoya. Mash the avocado with the chopped spinach and seeded, mashed cherimoya. *Absolutely delicious!*

Cherries

Even though cherries take a bit more work to eat than many fruits, with their hard little pits and rich, shirt-staining colors, they deserve special attention in your diet. They're a top source of perillyl alcohol—a compound that belongs to a group of compounds called monoterpenes. (Limonene, found in the peel of citrus fruits, is another member of this family.) These compounds have been shown in studies to block the formation of a variety of cancers, including those of the breasts, lungs, pancreas, stomach, liver, and skin. They've been demonstrated to kill cancer cells but spare healthy cells. Expectations for perillyl alcohol are high, in part because it's five to ten times more potent than limonene, which itself has been proven to be very effective.

Tart cherries, such as the best-known and most commercially grown Montmorency, contain significant amounts of melatonin, a hormone that helps normalize your sleep cycles. This substance also scavenges free radicals (unstable molecules that attack healthy cells), and having low levels of it has been linked to Alzheimer's disease. Cherries also contain a compound called quercetin. Like vitamin C and other antioxidants, it helps block the damage caused by free radicals. Studies show that quercetin may significantly reduce the risk of heart disease, stroke, and cancer.

Folklore is full of stories about people who relieved the agonizing pain of gout by eating cherries or drinking cherry juice daily. While the Arthritis Foundation says that there's no evidence to suggest that cherries really can ease the ache of gout, many sufferers swear by them. In fact, a survey by *Prevention* magazine found that 67 percent of readers who tried them had good results. In my holistic health practice, I've had success recommending this daily regimen: two to three glasses of black-cherry juice diluted with an equal amount of water, coupled with the elimination of all red and organ meats. For the best results, cut out *all* animal protein. In other words, become a vegan.

A dear friend who's a flight attendant shared a tip: She and her co-workers carry bags of dried cherries to help fight jet lag. When she told me this, I checked to see if there was any science behind it or if it was simply an old folktale. According to Dr. Russel Reiter, a nutrition researcher and one of the world's authorities on melatonin, it really might be true. "Tart cherries contain melatonin, which is then absorbed into the bloodstream, influencing your biological clock," he said. When flying east (say from Los Angeles to New York or New York to London), travelers should eat a handful of dried cherries (which have even greater levels of melatonin per pound than fresh ones) 30 minutes before trying to sleep.

Once at their destination, travelers should have a handful of cherries 30 minutes before going to bed every night for the same number of nights as the time change—that is, for a five-hour time shift, follow this regimen for five consecutive nights. When heading west, do the same thing, but begin the night before departure. Dr. Reiter added that concentrated cherry juice should have the same effect.

But there's more to this lush, juicy, tree-ripened fruit than exotic compounds. For example, sour cherries have voluminous quantities of vitamin C, along with iron, phosphorus, potassium, calcium, and vitamins A and E. Sweet cherries also contain these nutrients, but not as much vitamin A and E as the mouth-puckering variety. Because cooking destroys some of the vitamin C and other nutrients in the fruit, it's best to eat them raw to reap their full nutritional bounty. While you can find them frozen in your local natural-food store, I purchase several pounds of organic cherries when they're in season, pit them, and then dehydrate or freeze them so that I can enjoy their magnificence year-round.

Chicory

Chicory, also called "curly endive" or simply "endive," forms a loose bunch of ragged-edged leaves on long stems. A relative of Belgian endive and escarole, it's a member of the sunflower family. The outer leaves are deep green and have an assertive, slightly bitter taste; the leaves in the center are yellow and milder tasting. If you have a penchant for leafy green salads—one of the most nutritious meals you can eat—try adding some chicory to your bowl for its unique flavor and nutritional boon.

This plant has more vitamin A than any other salad green (just ¼ cup of raw chicory provides all of your recommended daily intake). The nutrient is essential for a healthy immune system and protects your vision; and in this NATURE-FOOD, most of it comes from beta-carotene, a cancer-fighting carotenoid that your body converts to vitamin A. Chicory leaves also are an excellent source of potassium and a good source of calcium and vitamin C. This bitter spring tonic food cleanses and helps regulate the liver and gallbladder. It purifies the blood, improves digestion, and nourishes the heart and circulatory system.

Chicory root, a popular ingredient in herbal coffees, contains an anticancer carbohydrate known as inulin, which prevented the formation of colon-cancer tumors in several animal studies, according to a review published in 2002 in the *British Journal of Nutrition*. Inulin also helps diabetics regulate their blood sugar levels.

There are numerous green and red chicories, which may be shaped like compact romaine or loose-leaf lettuce. Their leaves range from very narrow and highly serrated (frisée) to almost semicircular (radicchio). Look for fresh, crisp greens, and avoid those with wilting or browning.

Chlorella

Of all of the different types of green foods out there, only one has been around for 540 million years, making it the oldest living organism on Earth. Over ten million people around the world use chlorella every day to supplement their diets, and it's surely one of the most thoroughly researched foods of our time. Thousands of papers from many universities and medical schools around the world have been published on this topic, according to the late Dr. Bernard Jensen, nutritional expert and author of *Chlorella: Jewel of the Far East.*

A rich source of chlorophyll, chlorella is teeming with nutrients. Ounce for ounce, one gram gives you almost twice as much protein as soybean and almost eight times as much as rice. That's because chlorella contains more than 50 percent protein. It also has 18 vitamins and minerals and a complete range of amino acids. At the core of its purifying powers is a unique complex called *chlorella growth factor (CGF)*. All of the elements within the NatureFood's nucleus—peptides, proteins, nucleic acids, polysaccharides, and beta-glutens—combine to form CGF, which helps purify and remove toxins from the body, stimulate growth in children, repair damaged tissue, and boost the body's natural defense system. Research has shown that CGF is manufactured during the most intense periods of photosynthesis, incorporating within its structure the powerful energy of sunlight.

But with all of the different brands of chlorella out there—all claiming to be "the best"—how can you tell which one really will provide the greatest results and most health-boosting benefits? Let's take a look at the best pulverized chlorella on Earth.

Sun Chlorella is far superior to any other on the market. Compared to 34 other brands, it was the *only* one in which the hard outer cell wall was pulverized by an exclusive, patented technology called DYNO-Mill. Unlike the way other brands are produced, this company's process doesn't use heat or chemicals and thus is able to break down the hard outer cell wall so that it's 95 percent pulverized for maximum digestion and absorption, thereby providing the greatest results. Typical brands have an unbroken cell wall, which lacks the nutritional value of pulverized chlorella.

Also, Sun Chlorella uses the most powerful strain of *chlorella pyrenoidosa*. Compared to other strains in the world, Sun Chlorella's selected strain provides the richest source of CGF and other nutrients.

To give you an even better idea of the difference between the nutritional value gained from Sun Chlorella versus other brands, let's think of it in terms of the nutritional value found in fresh broccoli versus frozen. The bag you purchase from your supermarket's freezer section has less calcium, iron, thiamine, riboflavin, and vitamin C than the fresh stalks found in the produce section. So, while Sun Chlorella and other brands all may be producers of chlorella (similar to how fresh broccoli and frozen broccoli are both still broccoli), Sun Chlorella is superior in its CGF value and its patented DYNO-Mill pulverization process, thus allowing for far more absorption and digestibility of nutrients (much the way the fresh vegetable has greater nutritional value and benefits than the frozen variety).

Other brands also contain unwanted additives such as shellac, carnauba wax, stearic acid, silicon bioxide, cross carmellose sodium, acacia gum, and carboxy-methylcellulose in their products! Sun Chlorella is all-natural food and contains no artificial ingredients or additives. That's why I've taken it for more than 20 years. For more information or to order, please visit: **www.sunchlorellausa.com** or call: (800) 829-2828.

Chlorophyll

One thing that all green foods have in common is the fact that they contain varying levels of chlorophyll, which takes its name from the Greek *chloros,* meaning "yellowish green." It's the chemical that gives plants their green color. However, its function in nature is much more important than just appearances. Through the process of photosynthesis, chlorophyll helps convert the sun's energy into a form adequate for human and animal consumption and utilization.

Nearly identical to human blood, chlorophyll differs only in that it uses magnesium instead of iron as a bond. Chlorophyll contains virtually the full spectrum of minerals, vitamins, enzymes, and proteins.

"The actual chemical equation that takes place is the reaction between carbon dioxide and water, catalyzed by sunlight to produce glucose and a waste product, oxygen," according to Paul May, Ph.D., a senior lecturer in chemistry at the University of Bristol. "The glucose sugar is either directly used as an energy source by the plant for metabolism or growth, or it is polymerized to form starch so it can be stored until needed. The waste oxygen is excreted into the atmosphere, where it is made use of by plants and animals for respiration."

In addition to its essential function for sustaining much of the life on Earth, chlorophyll also may have protective effects against cancer. According to 2004 research published in *Methods in Molecular Biology,* chlorophyll—and its water-soluble derivative, chlorophyllin—are "potent inhibitors of carcinogenesis."

Several animal and in vitro studies have demonstrated these effects. Researchers at the Linus Pauling Institute at Oregon State University in Corvallis reported in the February–March 2003 issue of *Mutation Research* that chlorophyll and chlorophyllin suppressed abnormal cellular changes in an animal model of induced cancer. In the February 2004 issue of the same journal, researchers from the Universidade Estadual de Londrina in Brazil showed that chlorophyllin prevents damage to chemically treated cells.

In a human trial, oral chlorophyllin treatment three times per day was shown to potentially reduce the risk of liver cancer in a population at high risk for the disease due to aflatoxin exposure. Researchers who published their findings in the February–March 2003 issue of *Mutation Research* reported a 50 percent decline in the urinary excretion of an aflatoxin biomarker that seems to indicate a high risk for liver cancer.

While I could write an entire book on the benefits of chlorophyll to human health, suffice it to say that the more green foods you eat and drink, the healthier you'll be. Find ways to eat several servings of green foods daily. For example, I usually have two large green salads each day with a variety of both leafy greens and chopped green vegetables. I also make fresh green juices daily with several green vegetables and herbs, such as spinach, kale, collards, chard, parsley, celery, cucumber, and peppers, with some apple or carrot to sweeten them. I also mix a variety of super green grass powders into my water, teas, soups, or smoothies and take green supplement tablets on a regular basis. When you're green inside, you're clean and healthy inside. In my estimation, green foods are the most healthful ones you can eat, and you can never get too much.

(Refer to the recipes in this book as well as my books *The Healing Power of NatureFoods, Recipes for Health Bliss,* and *Be Healthy~Stay Balanced* for more green-food suggestions and lots of easy-to-prepare, tasty, and nutritious recipes.)

Collards

A mild-tasting variety of kale, collards are blue green with large, smooth, nonheading, paddle-like leaves. A favorite "soul" food of the American South, they're available 12 months of the year. This cruciferous vegetable with anti-cancer potential is among the oldest members of the cabbage family to have been cultivated. Collards are one of the milder greens; their flavor is somewhere between cabbage and kale. They provide potassium and contain nearly the same amount of calcium as milk, with approximately 226 mg in 3½ ounces raw (that's two to three cups). This amount also provides 23 mg of vitamin C, 0.6 mg of iron, and only a minuscule 19 calories.

Collards provide an incredibly nutritious roster of other nutrients and benefits. They're a heart-healthy food and one of the greens highest in carotenoids (along with spinach, beet and mustard greens, kale, and turnip and dandelion greens). Just ½ cup of cooked collards supplies 95 percent of a healthful daily intake of beta-carotene and 85 percent of the daily intake of lutein and zeaxanthin. These leaves also are an excellent source of folate, which plays a significant role in preventing cardiovascular disease and is one of the key nutrients in DNA repair.

It's not surprising that collards would be a powerful anticancer food, given the high level of nutrients and phytonutrients they contain. Glutathione and alpha lipoic acid are two antioxidants that researchers believe are the most important. Normally, these life-preserving nutrients are manufactured in the body itself, but our ability to produce them seems to diminish as we age. Collards contain a ready-made supply of both. Glutathione is the primary antioxidant in all cells, where its critically important job is to protect our DNA. It also repairs damaged DNA, promotes healthy cell replication, strengthens the immune system, detoxifies pollutants, and reduces chronic inflammation.

Alpha lipoic acid boosts glutathione levels by helping cells absorb a critical amino acid that's needed to make it. But there's more to this amazing phytonutrient, which is what I refer to as a "super-antioxidant." Most other antioxidants are soluble in either watery portions of the body (such as the blood) or fatty tissues (such as cell membranes). Alpha lipoic acid is soluble in both, meaning that it can help defend every type of substance in the body against oxidative assaults. It assists the body in breaking down sugar for energy production; it guards against strokes, heart attacks, and cataracts; it strengthens memory; and it turns off genes that can accelerate aging and cause cancer. That makes alpha lipoic acid a powerful nutrient for skin health, healing all types of damage—preventing skin cancer; restoring youthful vitality to the skin on your face, neck, and hands; and making your complexion more beautiful and youthful.

To prepare collards, wash the leaves first. If serving them in salads, dry them in paper towels or a salad spinner; if cooking, leave them damp. They can be blanched, braised, microwaved, sautéed, simmered, steamed, or (my favorite way to enjoy them) juiced and combined with other vegetables for a nutrient-rich "antioxidant elixir."

Corn

Indigenous to the western hemisphere, corn is the most abundant grain crop worldwide; it's exceeded only by wheat as a cereal grain. Purists claim the only way to cook corn on the cob is to have the water boiling before the corn is even picked because that's when the veggie is at its sweetest; the sugar starts turning to starch the instant it's plucked from the stalk. This NatureFood is best from May through September. Choose ears with husks that are tightly wrapped, grass green, and slightly damp. The silk can be dry, but shouldn't be rotting; stem ends need to be moist, not yellowed. It's best not to store the corn.

Popcorn is a field-type corn with thick-walled kernels; when heated, steam is trapped inside the dried kernels, causing them to "explode." Sweet corn—which wasn't widely cultivated until the mid-1800s—is harvested at an immature stage so that its kernels are tender and juicy. At their peak of flavor, sweet corn kernels contain 5–6 percent sugar by weight.

Maize, which many Americans mistakenly think is the Native American word for corn, is the term used for this vegetable in countries other than the United States. *Corn*, in those regions, denotes whatever happens to be the most popular cereal grain. In England, for example, "corn" refers to wheat, and in Scotland and Ireland, it signifies oats. Aside from feeding animals, the single largest industrial use of American corn is the production of sweeteners for beverages.

Versatile indeed, this food can be boiled, microwaved, roasted, steamed, popped, and grilled. Air-popped, unbuttered popcorn is low in calories and very high in fiber—a good snack for corn lovers. The veggie is also popular as cornmeal, which can be made into dishes such as corn bread and polenta. My favorite way to eat corn is simply to cut it raw right off the cob and sprinkle the kernels into my salads for an appealing crunch and color enhancement.

One of the best-balanced starches, fresh raw (or lightly steamed) corn is easy to digest. But after the grain has been dried, corn and corn cereals are some of the most difficult of all the cereals to digest. One medium ear contains about 85 calories. One cup of kernels provides 13 percent of the RDA for folate (the plant form of folic acid). It's also a source of potassium, thiamine, and fiber and is the only grain that contains vitamin A; yellow corn is higher in vitamin A than white corn. This multipurpose vegetable is a good source of lutein, a powerful antioxidant that may help lower the risk of age-related macular degeneration, a common cause of blindness in older adults.

Some of the latest research reveals that cooking sweet corn unleashes beneficial nutrients that can substantially reduce your risk of heart disease and cancer, according to a study in the *Journal of Agricultural and Food Chemistry*. The researchers found that the longer the corn was cooked, the higher the level of antioxidants. In addition to its antioxidant benefits, cooked sweet corn contains a phenolic compound called ferulic acid, which may inhibit cancer-causing substances. Corn oil is high in linoleic acid and also has fair amounts of oleic, linolenic, and arachidonic acids. The whole-grain oil has been found to correct over-alkalinity of the bodily system, and some doctors recommend it (either by the spoonful or applied directly to the skin) in cases of eczema-type skin disorders.

Except for being lower in vitamin C, canned and frozen corn are about equal in nutritional value to fresh corn. I favor fresh raw corn over frozen, and fresh frozen over canned. Canned corn usually has both salt and sugar added, making it marginally higher in calories and sometimes substantially higher in sodium than a similarly prepared fresh variety. And despite its name, canned "cream-style" corn has no milk or cream added; it's prepared with sugar and cornstarch, which further raise its calorie (but not its fat) content.

Daikon

Also called a Japanese or oriental radish, daikon is a large Asian radish with a peppery but sweet, fresh flavor. It's a bit hotter than red radishes but milder than black ones. I love its flavor, crisp texture, and great versatility. It's an easy— and rewarding—vegetable to grow due to its surprisingly hefty yield. These roots look like enormous white carrots (they grow to 18 inches). Once a stranger to the North American market, daikons have gained popularity recently.

Choose firm, smooth roots with a luminous white gleam. If they're an opaque, flat white, they've been stored too long. Because daikons don't keep well, they're best eaten within a day or two of purchase. Remove any attached greens, wrap in plastic, and refrigerate for up to three days.

Because the skin is thin, it generally doesn't need to be removed. Daikon can be cut into cubes or strips and stir-fried (in water). The way I use it the most, however, is for juicing, grating, adding to salads, or simply eating with a dip.

One of my favorite foods, this giant vegetable offers a powerhouse of health benefits. Fresh daikons contain diuretics; decongestants; and the digestive enzymes diastase, amylase, and esterase. They're effective against many bacterial and fungal infections, and they contain a substance that inhibits the formation of carcinogens in the body. If you're having any digestive problems, add three to four tablespoons of grated daikons to your meals throughout the day—especially the largest one that incorporates cooked food. Because the root aids digestion, in Japanese cuisine it often appears alongside hard-to-digest or fatty raw foods.

Daikons also support and help tone the liver and lungs. Phlegm in the lungs is often brought about by weak digestion that causes mucus, which can also result from too much mucus-forming food—especially an overabundance of cooked food, including dairy and other animal products. Either way, mucus accumulates in the lungs; symptoms include cough, shortness of breath, wheezing, or asthma accompanied by sticky phlegm. Daikon helps transform, reduce, or expel phlegm.

A dieter's best friend, one cup of fresh, sliced daikon has *only 15 calories,* one gram of protein, four grams of carbohydrates, and lots of salubrious enzymes.

Dandelion

You've probably seen it hundreds of times and thought this venerable herb was just a pesky weed. In spite of the plethora of herbicides that try to eliminate it, dandelion reigns indomitable on suburban lawns and byways. That gives some insight as to the heroism of this vegetable and the reason why the French and others esteem it.

In days gone by, lovers used the feathery seed balls of dandelions as oracles. Young maidens would blow three times on the fluff to determine if their sweethearts were thinking of them; the girl was not forgotten if a lone feather remained. Dandelion greens were so highly prized by the Apache that they would spend days or weeks searching the surrounding countryside for them. When I was a child, my mom and grandmother told me that if I made a wish while holding the stem and blowing off *all* of the fluff with one breath, the wish would come true. It's funny how I still make wishes this way!

Dandelions are of Eurasian origin, but today grow wild throughout the temperate world. The deeply notched leaves explain its Middle Latin name, *dent leo,* tooth of the lion. Perhaps the world's most famous weed, this ubiquitous plant is extremely hardy. Some believe that the dandelion will be among the few plants to survive all of the herbicides we've deposited on this planet. Although lawn owners feverishly dig it up, the plant actually heals the earth by transporting minerals (especially calcium) upward from deep layers, even from underneath hardpan. With this in mind, maybe you'll think twice about yanking out your garden's crops of dandelion.

Whether wild or cultivated, this NatureFood boasts a bounty of health benefits. A cup of dandelion greens provides nearly a day's requirement of vitamin

A in the form of the antioxidant carotenoid and a third of the daily vitamin C requirement. It contains more calcium than broccoli and is an excellent source of potassium, with very few calories (like all leafy greens).

Both the root and leaves of this herb are a remarkable (though bitter) tonic for the spleen, pancreas, kidney, stomach, and liver. (Other useful bitter herbs are chamomile and yellow dock root.) Dandelion is an efficacious diuretic; its French nickname *pissenlit* means "wet the bed." When clients ask me for an effective diuretic or laxative, for help reducing problems with premenstrual bloating, or for something to assuage rheumatism, I often recommend dandelion tea. It stimulates liver function, reduces swelling and inflammation, and improves digestion. And if that weren't enough, the plant is also antiviral and has been beneficial in the treatment of jaundice, cirrhosis, edema due to high blood pressure, gout, eczema, and acne. It's been found useful in the treatment of herpes, AIDS, breast and lung tumors, and hepatitis. Because dandelion root contains inulin, which lowers blood sugar, it's also highly recommended for diabetics.

I often enjoy salads made of tender, young dandelion leaves with vinaigrette dressing. Sometimes I combine them with other greens and flower blossoms for a panoply of color and taste sensations. The leaves can be steamed and seasoned with onion, vinegar, lemon, or herbs and served like spinach. Unopened buds are excellent nutlike morsels, delicious in salads and as a tea for indigestion.

Dandelion root has a stronger flavor than the highly cultivated vegetables/herbs most of us are accustomed to, with a marked taste that's both slightly sweet and bitter. Young roots are good chopped and added to salads; peeled and sautéed to be served as a tasty vegetable; or dried, roasted, and ground to be used as a caffeine-free coffee substitute.

So the next time you see a dandelion in your garden or during your pedestrian travels, instead of viewing it disdainfully, give it the respect it deserves.

Dark Chocolate

Whether during the holiday season or any other time of year, chocolate seems to be a ubiquitous favorite. I thought you'd appreciate learning about its benefits so you can savor every bite guilt free.

Cocoa, the main ingredient of chocolate, provides an impressive amount of antioxidant flavonoids, which fight heart disease and cancer. In a study published in *The American Journal of Clinical Nutrition* in 2001, 23 fortunate subjects added about four tablespoons of cocoa and about ½ ounce of dark chocolate daily to their average American diet. The additions improved their cholesterol ratios and increased the levels of antioxidants in their blood.

The plant chemicals in cocoa are also noteworthy. A recent preliminary study published in *The Cancer Letter* found that they prevented the growth of colon-cancer cells. In another study reported in the journal *Nature,* researchers analyzed blood samples from volunteers after they consumed dark chocolate, milk chocolate, and dark chocolate along with milk. One hour later, the dark chocolate significantly increased antioxidant levels. Milk, however, seemed to interfere with antioxidant absorption, rendering milk chocolate powerless against disease.

In 2007, a study published in *The Journal of the American Medical Association* discussed how just a small amount of dark chocolate, roughly one to two ounces, will help lower blood pressure and protect your heart. Keep in mind, however, that we're talking ounces, not pounds! And when you reach for this treat, make sure it's dark chocolate and choose the best quality possible. I usually look for an organic variety.

All chocolate comes from cacao beans (cacao nibs)—the seeds of the cacao fruit. Processing, cooking, and roasting malign the delicate, complex flavor of the cacao nib. *Raw* chocolate is a great source of antioxidants—20 times more than red wine, 30 times more than green tea. It's also rich in magnesium, chromium, and vitamin C. And unlike most candy, raw chocolate has a moderate glycemic index, which means that it provides steady energy instead of a sugar rush (and subsequent crash).

Of course, chocolate is high in fat and calories. To maximize your health benefits, choose dark chocolate (and raw sources whenever possible) and limit yourself to an ounce a day. I always have organic raw cocoa powder on hand and use it when making healthful smoothies or shakes, raw pie fillings and crusts, and chocolate syrups and sauces. You'll find a unique recipe for a Chocolate–Sweet Potato Smoothie in my book *The Healing Power of NatureFoods.* You can purchase raw, organic chocolate powder at your natural-food store.

I also use cacao nibs, blending them into my smoothie, tea, or favorite nutritional beverage; sprinkling them on my "ice cream" (frozen fruit) made in my Champion juicer; and adding them to any recipe instead of using chocolate chips. Kids love them, too! You'll find certified organic, raw chocolate (raw cacao nibs) in your natural-food store.

Dates

Prized for their sweet fruits, date palms are among the oldest cultivated trees; they've been grown in North Africa for at least 8,000 years. These desert dwellers are extraordinarily fruitful, producing up to 200 dates in a cluster.

If you've never experienced the sweetness of a date, a treat awaits you. The fruits have a papery-thin skin and a long, narrow seed surrounded by extremely sweet flesh. Their length varies from one to two inches, depending on the variety. Their color also varies when ripe, from golden to deep brown. Fresh dates are available from late summer through mid-fall.

Choose fruits that are plump and soft, with a smooth, shiny skin. Avoid shriveled, moldy, or crystallized dates. Excessive shriveling; a dry, flaky appearance; or a fermented aroma indicates that they're old or have been improperly stored. Soft, fresh dates should be refrigerated or frozen; they can be stored in an airtight container for up to one year in the refrigerator and for up to five years in the freezer. They'll become drier in the refrigerator over time, while frozen dates have almost no loss in quality. Dried dates store indefinitely at room temperature.

These gems are nourishing and sweet and, unlike refined sweeteners, are teeming with nutritional gifts. One-half cup (about 12 medium dates) contains about 275 calories—many more than most fruits, but they also provide a wealth of potassium (650 mg), which is more than a comparable amount of other high-potassium foods, such as bananas and oranges. This portion also delivers iron, niacin, and vitamin B_6, as well as six grams of fiber. One of the drawbacks of dates is their high sugar content and stickiness, which promote tooth decay, so it's important to brush your teeth and use a Hydro Floss (see the Resources section) after eating them.

Based on the degree of dehydration, dates are classified in one or more of the following four types:

— **Fresh:** The *bahri* date is an example of this variety, and while not exactly juicy, it's higher in moisture content and lower in sugar content than other dates.

— **Soft:** Allowed to dry in the sun on the tree, soft dates, usually the *medjool* and *khadrawy* varieties, are then hydrated with steam to plump them back up. Medjools are my favorite dates; they hold an esteemed place in my freezer and refrigerator, and I use them most often as sweeteners in my smoothies and other culinary dishes. Regarded by many as the best-tasting type, the medjool is known for its impressive size, up to an ounce or more in weight, and is often many times larger than the *deglet noor.*

— **Semidry:** Because of their low moisture, these dates have a long shelf life and are available year-round. The *deglet noor* variety, which means "light of day," accounts for 85 percent of domestic production. Other varieties include *halawy* and *zahidi.*

— **Dry:** The least sticky and the driest variety, the *thoory* is often referred to as the bread date. With a firm skin and chewy flesh, it's a staple in the diet of nomadic Middle Eastern peoples.

Dates can be used as a sweetener, stuffed with an almond or other nut or nut butter and rolled in coconut (children love these), or added to many dishes—such as fruit salads, cereals, puddings, and baked goods, often substituting for raisins or currants. I also use date sugar. This is composed of 100 percent pitted dehydrated (3–5 percent moisture) dates that are coarsely ground; it's usually made from cosmetically inferior dates. With about 65 percent fructose and sucrose, if consumed in excess, it upsets the blood-sugar balance just as white sugar does. But used in moderation, date sugar is a quality sweetener, definitely more natural and unrefined than most, and it contains all of the nutrients of dried dates. You can sprinkle it on top of foods such as cereal, yogurt, or baked goods (added after baking to prevent burning), and you can dissolve date sugar in hot water to make a syrup similar to honey, maple syrup, or rice syrup.

Evening Primrose

Evening primrose (I love the name!) is a tiny, short-lived, bright yellow wildflower native to North America. After discovering this New World plant, Europeans took it back home, where its healing properties for skin diseases and flesh wounds quickly earned it the name "King's Cure-All." Currently, evening primrose is grown in 30 or more countries, and the oil pressed from its seed is marketed as a valuable natural-healing supplement. It's especially well documented for supporting skin health in cases of eczema and dermatitis. Other benefits include relief for arthritis-related joint pain and assuagement of premenstrual syndrome and symptoms of menopause such as cramps, hot flashes, breast tenderness, and moodiness.

Today, we know that the oil from the seeds of evening primrose contains a high amount of the active ingredient gamma-linolenic acid (GLA), which is quite similar to other essential fatty acids (EFA) of the omega-6 variety. In fact, evening-primrose oil is one of the few substances found in nature that contains significant amounts of GLA, which aids the body's formation of important prostaglandins (the prostaglandin E1 series, known as PGE1) that moderate inflammatory processes. (Prostaglandins are molecules that act as vital cell regulators.)

While the body manufactures gamma-linolenic acid from linoleic acid (one of the essential fatty acids), optimal production is often inhibited by dietary deficiencies, age-related enzymatic deficiencies, and consuming excess amounts of saturated fat. Indeed, it's interesting to note that linoleic acid has little or no biological activity in and of itself; its true value is in its conversion to GLA. When we take additional GLA, we encourage increased formation of PGE1, which produces a variety of health benefits.

Health experts say the prostaglandin E1 series aids the body by inhibiting or reducing inflammation, blood clumping, blood clots, abnormal cholesterol production, and formation of malignant cells. (In particular, GLA reduces risk of arterial spasm and abnormal clots, important factors in heart attacks and stroke.) Another benefit is lowering blood pressure. The PGE1 series also maintains important electrolyte balances and normalizes insulin secretions.

Other health conditions that benefit from gamma-linolenic acid include arthritis; skin disorders such as eczema, acne, and dermatitis; allergies and asthma; premenstrual syndrome; multiple sclerosis; fibrocystic breast disease; and depression.

In a small study from the department of dermatology, College of Medicine, University Republic of Korea, evening-primrose oil was given to dermatitis patients whose condition was characterized by itchy, dry, scaly skin. "After the treatment, the extent of the skin lesions and the pruritus were markedly reduced in all patients," noted researchers. They asserted that evening-primrose oil is "highly effective" in the treatment of a noninflammatory dermatitis. (Yoon, S., et al. "The therapeutic effect of evening primrose oil in atopic dermatitis patients with dry scaly skin lesions is associated with the normalization of serum gamma-interferon levels." *Skin Pharmacol Appl Skin Physiol*, 2002; 15(11): 20–25.)

Numerous other studies also show the effectiveness of evening-primrose oil for a wide range of conditions. It has been used to reduce cholesterol and blood pressure, help rheumatoid arthritis and similar inflammatory ailments, make withdrawal easier in alcoholism, relieve some of the distressing symptoms of multiple sclerosis, boost the immune system, and assist in weight control. In some cases of obesity, this substance may help by stimulating brown fat tissue to burn up calories and rectify metabolic abnormalities. Regular use of evening-primrose oil also might assist AIDS sufferers, with alleviation of skin sores and fatigue being among the reported benefits.

So if you're looking for an excellent natural supplement to support most primary body functions, promote healthy hormone levels, and aid the body's inflammation response, evening-primrose oil is perfect. Always look for a certified organic source—most consumers don't know that many types of oils tend to accumulate pesticide residues, especially from toxic, fat-soluble chemicals. In addition, since oils are highly subject to rancidity, it's recommended that you acquire a product that's manufactured using a low-temperature process without chemical solvents to avoid formation of free radicals and ensuing rancidity.

My favorite top-quality evening-primrose oil is made by Barlean's. The recommended amount is 2,600 milligrams per day, with higher doses of four to six grams recommended for conditions such as arthritis, asthma, or eczema. It's available in finer health-food stores nationwide.

Fennel

A member of the parsley family, fennel is also known as sweet fennel; Florence fennel; and, in Italian neighborhoods, *finocchio.* Europeans, particularly the Italians and the French, have been enthusiastic about this plant for many years. They cultivate more of it than anyone else, but the vegetable is becoming more widely appreciated in the United States. Similar to celery in looks, calories, and crunch, it's filling yet very low in calories, so it's an excellent snack food for those who are watching their weight. It's also well suited to baking, braising, roasting, sautéing, and steaming. I use it often when juicing and as a raw snack food.

Through the ages, physicians have used and venerated this vegetable for a variety of ailments. Hippocrates recommended fennel tea to stimulate milk production in nursing mothers. In India, ayurvedic physicians have long suggested fennel seeds to aid digestion and prevent bad breath. Nicholas Culpeper, the 17th-century British herbalist, used the plant to treat kidney stones, gout, and liver and lung disorders, and as an antidote to poisonous mushrooms. It's also one of the oldest diet remedies. Ancient Greek and Roman healers prescribed the seeds to prevent obesity; more modern herbalists advocate fennel tea as a diet aid.

The plant's flavor is sweeter and more delicate than anise, but because of its taste, it's called "anise" in many markets. However, the vegetable is an entirely different plant from the herb anise, which is grown for its seeds and the oil secreted by its leaves (both of which are used as flavorings). When cooked, fennel's flavor becomes even more mellow. The bulb, stalks, and flowery greens are all edible. The seeds, used for flavor, come from a nonbulbous fennel.

Choose clean, crisp, pearly bulbs with no sign of browning, and check for cracks. The attached greenery should be soft, fragrant, and green. Fennel doesn't store well. Wrap it tightly in a container and refrigerate for up to four or five days.

High in fiber like celery, one cup of fennel has only 25 calories. More nutritious than celery, it's brimming with vitamins A and C, iron, calcium, potassium, and more. The aromatic seeds are one of our oldest spices, and they're used to make a refreshing tea that's said to alleviate bloating, flatulence, and other intestinal problems. You can chew the leaves, bulb, or seeds for a pleasant, refreshing taste and breath sweetener. Fennel has a specific affinity for the bloodstream and builds strong plasma. If I've eaten a high-fat meal, I'll usually drink fennel tea while at the table or afterward because it helps accelerate the digestion of fatty foods.

Fermented Foods

The process of fermenting foods to preserve them and to make them more digestible and more nutritious is as old as humanity. We've been enjoying them for millennia—bread, coffee, chocolate, beer, wine, cheese, miso, yogurt, and sauerkraut are a few of the most familiar—relying on the magic of fermentation to preserve and enhance the flavor and health benefits of what we eat and drink. Fermented food is literally alive with complex bacterial activity so necessary to life itself.

In our haste to adopt newer, more technological food production, we've abandoned the fermenting that benefited our ancestors. Captain Cook, the 18th-century English explorer, set sail on a 27-day voyage with 60 barrels of sauerkraut to feed his crew. Throughout that journey, not one sailor suffered from the muscle weakness and spongy gums associated with scurvy, a common ailment of seafarers brought on by a severe vitamin C deficiency. As reported in an article in the magazine *Hallelujah Acres Diet & Lifestyle,* the fermentation of the sauerkraut increases the already naturally high content of vitamin C in the cabbage.

If you do an Internet search on the fermentation process, you'll discover thousands of Websites detailing everything from the "fun" of fermenting to various recipes to detailed scientific facts. The best book I've ever read on the subject is called *Wild Fermentation: The Flavor, Nutrition, and Craft of Live-Culture Foods,* by Sandor Ellix Katz. Comprehensive and enthralling, this book offers sensational recipes for fermented and live-culture cuisine. Much more than a cookbook, it's a "cultural manifesto" that explores the history and politics of human nutrition.

It's not difficult to ferment foods. For example, raw vegetables are cut, ground, or shredded and left in a covered sanitary container made of stainless steel, ceramic, or glass for about seven days at room temperature, between 50 and 71 degrees. The longer the vegetables steep, the stronger the taste. This process lets the beneficial flora, such as lactobacillus plantarum, go to work, breaking down the inherent sugars and starches in the vegetables.

Later in this book, you'll learn more about miso, a fermented food made from soybeans. It's uniquely grounding, and in Japanese folk wisdom, it has been long associated with good health and longevity. I enjoy miso as part of my healthful diet and use it in dressings, sauces, soups, and dips.

Every season or so, I make fresh batches of sauerkraut. In fact, I keep a few crocks of different types of ferments going for variety. Whether composed of just cabbage or a variety of plants, fermented vegetables complement any meal. Their tangy flavors accent the rest of the food, cleanse the palate, and improve digestion. I've used a panoply of vegetables in my culture and culinary classes. Some of my favorite ones to ferment are beets, cabbage, carrots, cauliflower, garlic, green beans, celery, leeks, kale, parsnips, carrots, radishes, rutabaga, shallots, turnips, kelp, and various herbs.

The main difference between vegetables left to rot and those destined for delicious fermentation is usually salt. The process is best under the protection of brine, which is simply water with salt dissolved in it. In some ferments, such as sauerkraut, the salt is used to draw water out of the vegetables, thus creating intense vegetable-juice brine. In other ferments, such as cucumber pickles, a brine solution is mixed and then poured over the vegetables.

Brine serves as protection against the growth of putrefying microorganisms and favors the growth of the desired strains of bacteria, *Lactobacilli*. The amount of salt (I use Celtic Sea Salt brand) in brine can vary considerably. The more you use, the slower the fermentation will be and the sourer (more acidic) the resulting ferment.

With too much salt, however, no microorganism can survive, and fermentation won't occur.

Kombucha is a fermented sour tonic beverage similar to rejuvelac (a slightly fermented wheat berry drink) and kvass (a slightly alcoholic beverage of eastern Europe made from fermented mixed cereals and often flavored). It's sweetened black tea, cultured with a "mother," also known as "the tea beast," a gelatinous colony of bacteria and yeast. The mother ferments the sweet tea and reproduces itself, like kefir grains. For more than ten years, I made my own fresh kombucha every week and only stopped because of my traveling schedule. Fortunately, I now can purchase deliciously flavored kombucha drinks in natural-food stores. This beverage is known to help rejuvenate, detoxify, and balance all of the body systems.

The scientific studies disclose that fermented foods help us detoxify, fight infections, reduce high cholesterol levels, and support the digestive and immune systems. Additionally, cultured foods are known to be a terrific source of amino acids, vitamins, and minerals, particularly B vitamins and omega-3 fatty acids.

Because the fermentation process can't take place without the active participation of live enzymes and bacteria, these foods are, in effect, probiotics that promote the growth of healthy flora and increase digestive enzymes, lactase, lactic acid, and other chemicals that battle harmful bacteria. As highlighted in the *Hallelujah Acres Diet & Lifestyle* article, fermented foods also act as antioxidants and might even help prevent and fight cancer.

If you're looking for ways to improve your digestion and enrich your health and vitality, add some fermented foods to your diet. You'll love what you taste and how you feel.

Flower Blossoms

Flowers not only delight the soul and add beauty to our homes, yards, and environments; they also can be a bright accompaniment to salads and other dishes. Their fragrance and essential oils, which are related to warmth, add a magical warming touch to a meal—the blossom's inner temperature is higher than the temperature outside. Colorful flower blossoms elicit a pause and then a deep breath. They rejuvenate the soul and somehow make the entire meal taste better.

The culinary use of flowers dates back thousands of years; the first recorded mention was 140 years before the Christian era. These days, it seems to be more popular than ever, especially in better restaurants. I often use blossoms in my food preparation simply because I like the beauty and splendor they exude.

There are a few simple guidelines that are important to consider when selecting flowers for culinary use. Foremost, be sure to use only edible blossoms that have been grown without the use of pesticides or other chemical sprays—in other words, only consume organic blossoms. Flowers from your local florist are generally treated, so those aren't the ones to select. If you have an organic home garden, that would be a great resource. To sensitive individuals, some blossoms may cause allergic reactions; moreover, some are poisonous. Don't eat Oriental lilies, lilies of the valley, sweet peas, or any of the narcissus family (daffodils, narcissus, paperwhites, and jonquils).

Pick your flowers in the morning, and rinse them quickly under gently running cool water. A good rule of thumb is to not gather more than what you'll use in a day, as the blossoms wilt quickly. And before using them in any preparation, remove the pistils, stamens, and the white part at the base of the petals; this "heel" will impart a bitter flavor to the finished dish.

Most edible flowers have a taste similar to their smell and are used mainly raw in salads or as a garnish. Because flavors differ from variety to variety, always taste them before use. For example, some roses are exquisitely sweet and others sour, metallic, or bitter. Some small- and medium-size blossoms are used whole. Unless stuffed, large blossoms—like the nasturtium or squash—may be sliced or torn. Susan Belsinger, author of *Flowers in the Kitchen,* recommends stuffing nasturtiums with guacamole for stellar flavor, color, and texture.

Edible flowers include:

— **Decorative flowers:** Possibilities include carnation, chrysanthemum, daisy, daylily, fuchsia, geranium (scented), gladiolus, hibiscus, hollyhock, honeysuckle, Johnny-jump-up, lavender, lilac, marigold (caution—sometimes very bitter), nasturtium, pansy, pinks, rose, viola, and violet. (Avoid daffodils and tulips because some may be toxic.)

— **Fruit blossoms:** All edible fruits have blossoms that you can eat: Apple, peach, plum, and lemon are all fragrant and delicately flavored. Orange, cherry, and strawberry flowers are a special delicacy.

— **Herb blossoms:** You may want to choose from bee balm, borage, calendula, chamomile, chive, dandelion, dill, garlic, marjoram, mint, mustard flowers, oregano, rosemary, savory, and thyme.

— **Vegetable blossoms**: All flowers of the cabbage, bean, and gourd families are edible. These include arugula, bean, chicory, cucumber, pea, and squash. Blooms can be picked from any squash, summer or winter variety, and zucchini plants produce particularly luxuriant ones.

"The art of healing comes from nature,
not from the physician.
Therefore the physician must start from nature,
with an open mind."

— PARACELSUS

PART III

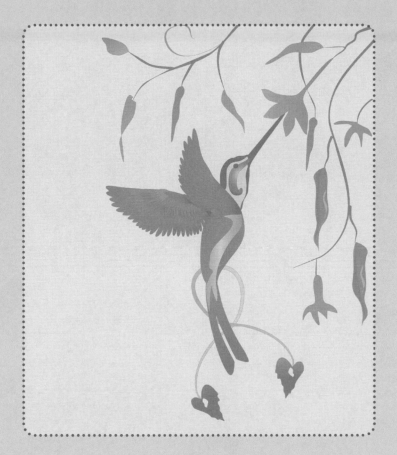

INTERMISSION

THE HEALING POWER
OF DEEP BREATHING

*"Live every moment, every hour, every day,
tranquilly in the protective love of God."*

— WHITE EAGLE

W hen several hundred participants in a stress-reduction workshop I gave (titled *BE HEALTHY~STAY BALANCED: 10 Simple Ways to Create More Joy & Less Stress*) were asked to name the most important thing they learned, the majority said "breathing." This may sound odd, since we all know how to breathe or we wouldn't be living. Yet in reality, these people found out that they didn't breathe *efficiently*. Once they learned to be more aware of this vital element, they found that stress had noticeably less impact on them. By simply helping them become more mindful of their breathing, I got them back in touch with the most basic of bodily functions.

How often do you pause to consider the intricacies of breathing? How much thought have you given to its impact on various aspects of your being? It's perhaps the only physiological process that can be either voluntary or involuntary. You can breathe "on command," making your breath do whatever you wish; or you can ignore it, allowing your body to simply go ahead on its own. When you do this, it becomes reflexive.

Your body can't operate without breathing, so if conscious control is abandoned, something is triggered in the unconscious part of the brain that does the work for you. During the periods of time when this is happening (which is almost always for most people), your breathing falls under the control of primitive parts of your brain, the unconscious realms where emotions, thoughts, and feelings (of which we may have little or no awareness) become involved. These wreak havoc with rhythms. In other words, the breath becomes haphazard and often irregular if you lose conscious control. It's important to bring breath back into your awareness so that it's reintegrated into your consciousness.

Thoracic Park

Are your breaths rapid and shallow? Take a minute now to check and see how many you take per minute. If your number is between 16 and 20 (count both the inhalation and exhalation as one breath), then you're most likely a thoracic breather. This means that the air isn't getting to the lower part of your lungs, but remaining fairly high in the chest. This is the least efficient and most common type.

Like bad eating habits, improper breathing patterns are mostly learned and culturally influenced. Have you ever been told to "suck in" your stomach? Both males and females in Western culture have incurred this "flat stomach" admonition, contributing to tight diaphragm muscles and restricted breathing.

The constant state of stress and imbalance in which many people live also promotes tightening of the abdominal muscles. Continual low-level fear or anxiety (fostered by commercial interests and their media outlets) contributes to a pattern of shallower, more rapid breathing, which results in insufficient oxygen reaching the brain. When this happens, you may feel unfocused and maybe even light-headed or dizzy. This pattern of thoracic breathing has a tendency to keep the fight-or-flight response in a constant state of readiness.

Cultivating the Habit of Deep Breathing

Diaphragmatic or deep abdominal breathing promotes a more relaxed state. Take a long, slow, deep breath right now. Visualize the air filling the lower part of the lungs. Since gravity pulls more blood into that area, the most efficient passage of oxygen into the blood occurs there, slowing the breath as the body gets more oxygen. As the breath slows (to six to eight breaths per minute) and deepens, the heart's job is made considerably easier. There is evidence to suggest that diaphragmatic breathing is beneficial because it increases the suction pressure created in the thoracic cavity and improves the venous return of blood, thereby reducing the load on the heart and enhancing circulatory function. It has the added bonus of relaxing the muscles of the ribs, chest, and stomach.

Diaphragmatic breathing is really quite simple, but it's important to consciously cultivate it as a habit so that it becomes automatic. A simple way to practice is to lie down on your back on a mat or rug, with one palm placed on the center of the chest and the other on the lower edge of the rib cage where the abdomen begins. As you inhale, the lower edge of the rib cage should expand and the abdomen should rise; as you exhale the opposite should occur. There should be relatively little movement of the upper chest. If you do this regularly, over time you will find that the method becomes habitual and automatic.

In order to make deep breathing the default pattern in my life, I tried this experiment several years ago. I set my watch to beep every hour (except when I was sleeping, of course), and I took one to three minutes to do some deep breathing. As the days and weeks went on, I noticed that when the hourly beep came around, I was already practicing deep breathing; it was becoming a habit. Now, most of the time, it's my natural response.

Harmonious, Rhythmic Breathing

Adopting the habit of harmonious and rhythmic breathing—observing the rate of breaths per minute on both inhalation and exhalation—along with diaphragmatic breathing is highly therapeutic and not at all difficult. Start by slowing down the inhalation because that's affected by nerve centers, the diaphragm, and the intercostal and abdominal muscles. Plasma from the capillaries moves out into the alveolar space during inhalation and moves back into the capillaries during exhalation. During this process, nutrients from the blood ooze out into the air sacs, where they're acted upon by enzymes and made available for your body to use. Lengthening inhalation increases time for this metabolic function to take place.

Rhythmic diaphragmatic breathing also brings more air and oxygen into the air sacs of the lungs and into the bloodstream. It increases the return of venous blood to the lungs and sends an increased blood supply to the capillaries of the alveoli. In addition, since the pericardium is attached to the diaphragm, the process of deep breathing causes the diaphragm to descend, stretching the heart downward toward the abdomen. When the lungs are filled with air from the bottom upward, they compress, giving a gentle massage to the heart. As the diaphragm contracts and relaxes, it also massages the heart, liver, and pancreas and helps improve the functions of spleen, stomach, small intestine, and abdomen, as well.

Deep breathing can be practiced while standing, sitting, or lying on your back with your arms by your sides, palms upward, and legs slightly apart. Exhalation should be through the nostrils, and there should be no external sound. Having exhaled completely, begin inhalation, minimizing the pause, again using the nostrils and making no external sound. Gradually, increase the length of time of each inhalation and exhalation. If you practice rhythmic diaphragmatic breathing just ten times each day for at least two months, you'll experience deep rest and relaxation and remain free from stress and strain. Your nerves will be calm, your voice will relax, and your face will shine with a soft, healthy glow.

A Healthier, More Energized Life Is a Few Breaths Away

Another efficacious way to more fully oxygenate your body is through a superlative device called *Activated Air* by Eng[3]. As you age, your cells' ability to effectively use the oxygen in the air you breathe diminishes, even if you practice deep breathing on a regular basis. I highly recommend Activated Air—a salutary breathing therapy that will optimize your oxygen supply and make a positive difference in how you feel. Developed by European scientists, Activated Air helps you keep your cellular energy production in top shape. Maximizing the cells' ability to produce energy is the best protection against illness and the effects of aging. It improves your overall health and quality of life, retards age-related diseases and disorders, reduces damage from excess free radicals, enhances cellular regeneration, maximizes your ability to draw nutrition from your food, improves athletic performance, and shortens recovery time.

While oxygen therapy such as that found in oxygen bars will give you a temporary boost in energy, it has no long-term positive effect on your health. Activated Air, on the other hand, improves your body's ability to use the oxygen you're already breathing and cuts down on free-radical pollution that doctors say causes a variety of diseases and premature aging. It's completely natural and contains no chemicals or drugs of any kind; it's the best way I know to help make oxygen more available to your cells. It's completely safe and can be combined with other treatments.

My policy always has been to recommend only those products that I use personally or recommend to my friends and clients—products that I consider to be the best of the best. I've seen noticeable, positive differences in how I look and feel and how my clients feel after using Activated Air. I now sleep better, have an easier time concentrating and focusing on my work, exercise harder without tiring, recover more rapidly, have more energy than ever, and enjoy many other noticeable benefits.

If you're interested in losing weight, definitely consider purchasing an Activated Air. With maximized oxygen uptake, you use fat more easily as your body's fuel source. In other words, you'll have an easier time losing weight—you'll experience an acceleration of fat loss, especially when combined with optimal diet and regular exercise.

Activated Air is FDA approved and is easy to use in the privacy of your home or office—I even take it with me (in its own carrying case) when I travel. Simply sit back, relax, and breathe through the nasal attachment. I use it most often when watching TV, working at my computer, and meditating. Some of my clients use it when sleeping. Your pets also can reap the benefits of this simple device. All this for just 20 minutes per day, three days a week.

Please refer to: **www.SusanSmithJones.com** and click on *Susan's Favorite Products* for a more detailed write-up on Activated Air and why I recommend it to everyone. If you have additional questions, visit: **www.eng3corp.com** or call toll-free: (877) 571-9206. A healthier, happier, and more energized life could be just a few breaths away.

❋ ✻ ❋

The Healing Power of Neti: Nasal Cleansing

*"You can accomplish anything if you do not accept limitations. . . .
Whatever you make up your mind to do, you can do."*

— PARAMAHANSA YOGANANDA

When I was 18, I learned about the healing power of *neti*—nasal cleansing—from my grandmother, Fritzie. At that time in my life, my diet was deplorable. Meat, sweets, and white refined-flour breads were my daily pleasures, and my health sorely suffered as a result. I was rarely without allergies, and I carried copious amounts of tissues with me everywhere to wipe my runny nose, deal with my sneezing, and take care of all the extra mucus that I was coughing up. It wasn't a pretty picture, and my physician informed me that I would have to live with this condition for the rest of my life.

When my grandmother heard about what the doctor said, she took me aside and gave me sage advice that I've never forgotten. She said that if I followed her instructions 100 percent, she guaranteed that my allergies and sinus problems would resolve within 30 days and that my entire life would change profoundly for the better. She predicted that my acne would clear up, my energy would soar, the extra weight I was carrying would fall away, and my attitude would change from negative to positive. Needless to say, she had my attention.

Over the next several hours, I learned a variety of health practices that—although they sounded odd to me at that time—touched a responsive chord in my heart. The well-known adage "When the student is ready, the teacher will appear," was definitely true for me. I was ready, and with my grandmother's ongoing, loving support, my entire life began to change for the better. Along with a new diet of natural, whole foods; deep breathing; visualization; meditation; and other practices, she introduced me to neti.

Fritzie called this her "easy breathing" practice. She didn't have a neti pot; she used a small teapot with a spout. In less than four weeks of practicing nasal cleansing two times each day (in addition to meditating, visualizing, and eating my new diet), I was free from excess mucus, allergies, sneezing, constant throat clearing, extra weight, and my former pessimistic attitude. My grandmother went from being someone whose "health nut" approach to life seemed strange to me to being my greatest mentor—the person who changed my life for the better. The things she taught me in the years before she passed are among the greatest blessings and life lessons I ever received, and I teach them to this day. Based on her guidance, I chose my life career; my passion for alternative and holistic health was born.

Time-Tested Practice

The simple practice of nasal irrigation known as neti has been used by practitioners of yoga and ayurveda in India for more than 5,000 years. The term *neti,* which originally meant "to guide," refers to the water that moves energy through the nasal passages, opening them up along the way. Nasal cleansing isn't simply an ancient health secret; doctors, naturopaths, and other health professionals recommend it today. This salutary, time-tested practice of personal hygiene can benefit almost everyone, and neti pots are now available in natural-food stores and herbal shops around the country and worldwide.

Some yogic teachers consider neti valuable in cleansing the energy channels and balancing the right and left hemispheres to create radiant, energetic health and wellness. Dr. Andrew Weil, among others, is a strong proponent of nasal cleansing on a regular basis. Research and articles have appeared in a number of professional journals such as the *Academy of Otolaryngology.* Research conducted at Harvard Medical School shows that nasal cleansing can aid in various chronic and acute conditions, including allergic rhinitis and acute sinusitis. Doctors and alternative-health practitioners around the world recommend the routine practice of nasal cleansing using a saline solution as part of a regular regimen of health and well-being.

Put simply, while the practice of nasal irrigation may have originated in India, today there are large numbers of people in Europe and North America who have added this simple technique to their daily hygiene. Many individuals practice neti on a daily basis to keep their sinuses clean and improve their ability to breathe freely, and most find it a soothing and pleasant practice once they try it.

How's Your Breathing?

Have you ever suffered from not being able to breathe fully through both nostrils, even when you didn't have a cold? Have you ever wished there was a way to just pour some soothing warm water through your nose to remove all of the extra mucus? Even if you rarely suffer from sinus or nasal problems, you've probably experienced a dry or clogged nose in environments with low humidity, such as in the cabin of an airplane or during Santa Ana winds that are common in Southern California. Or maybe you live in an environment where the air isn't clean—where there's pollution from chemicals, smog, and diesel residues, or secondhand cigarette smoke. Some people are even sensitive to household products, fragrances, and other synthetic odors, as well as dust and pollen. All of these irritants stimulate your body's production of nasal mucus as a natural process to protect and help cleanse the nasal passages.

In addition to the discomfort that comes from external sources, the nose and nasal passages are equally sensitive to internal irritations, such as those that arise as a result of eating mucus-forming foods. The standard American diet (SAD) is fraught with ingredients that increase mucus in the body, and one of the primary places that excess accumulates is the head. Foods that cause an increase in mucus include dairy products, pastries, breads, sweets, unhealthful fats (such as trans and hydrogenated), and fried items of all types. Things that are greasy, sweet, or highly salted also tend to increase mucus, as does a diet that consists mostly or entirely of cooked food. When you have excess mucus in your sinuses and throughout your head from unhealthful choices, it impairs your breathing.

Excess mucus also increases as a result of a sedentary lifestyle because lack of movement contributes to poor circulation. When blood flow is impeded, whether due to lack of exercise or sitting too many hours at your desk, it can lead to stagnation in the body and the mind that allows toxins and mucus to build up. And if you combine a diet of high mucus-forming foods with exposure to polluted air, this problem will be exacerbated.

If you're one of the many people who find that your nasal passages are blocked as a result of the effects of your diet, pollution, dust, pollen, and other irritants, you may find the following simple cleansing technique of invaluable benefit to you. While there are advanced methods using various herbs and herbal oils, the simplest option—and the one I practice most often—uses lukewarm water for the cleansing process. It's a gentle means of opening up the nasal passages.

A Natural, Easy Practice

It seems so natural to me to practice nasal cleansing daily, and I even take my small neti pot with me when I travel. While I sometimes go through my routine twice each day, the morning is my favorite time, and it's part of my personal hygiene ritual: I brush and floss my teeth, scrape my tongue, and cleanse out my nasal passages. I prefer doing this early in the day because mucus accumulates in the head during the night, and congestion often develops as a result. It's important to clear this out first thing so that there's a proper flow of energy for the rest of the day.

But it's also beneficial to use the neti pot before sleep to ensure that the nasal passages are open for optimal breathing as you rest. This prevents snoring and mouth breathing and can help you enjoy deeper, more relaxing sleep.

In addition to personally doing nasal irrigation for decades, I highly recommend it to clients in my private practice. I especially advise it for anyone with sinus problems and environmental allergies. Within 30–90 days of practicing neti once or twice daily, I've seen many clients and friends heal their sinusitis and eliminate the need for allergy medications (even those who had been on such drugs for years).

How to Keep Your Nose Clean

Here's my daily nasal-cleansing process: Mix approximately ¼ teaspoon of fine sea salt into about one cup (eight ounces) of warm water until it's fully dissolved. The water should be warm, but not hot. It should feel pleasantly warm to the touch so as not to irritate your nasal passages. You may prefer to use bottled water if your local water supply is too hard or has chemicals or an unappealing taste.

Next, pour your saline solution into the nasal-cleansing pot. Tilt your head to the side. Insert the spout gently into the raised (upper) nostril and create a seal between the pot and your nostril. Don't be afraid to adjust your head slightly to get the most comfortable angle for your own personal practice. You'll probably discover that having your forehead on about the same level as your chin will be just right.

Raise the nasal-cleaning pot slowly to develop a steady flow of saline solution through the upper nostril and out the lower one. You're in total control of the stream by the way you hold the pot—the higher you hold it, the faster the flow.

During the process, you breathe through your mouth. The angle of your head is important to allow you to breathe easily through your mouth. Upon completion, exhale gently through your nose several times to clear the nasal passages. You may want to use a tissue to catch any excess mucus.

Reverse the tilt of your head and repeat the process on the other side. I usually can clear both sides with one pot full of saline solution, but some people prefer using an entire potful for each nostril. Once you get into practice, the entire cycle only takes a couple of minutes.

It's beneficial to do some simple, gentle exhalation—blowing through both of your nostrils—after you're finished. Either do this over a sink or into a tissue. Be sure to not close off your nostrils as you blow, because you want to expel the excess solution and any residual mucus.

After use, simply wash out the pot with warm water and dish soap, and thoroughly rinse away all soap and other residues. The nasal pot that I recommend is made out of sturdy food-grade porcelain so that it's dishwasher safe.

Some of the many benefits of using the nasal-cleansing pot include the following:

- ✳ Clears the nostrils to free the breathing
- ✳ Removes excess mucus
- ✳ Reduces pollen or allergens in the nasal passages
- ✳ Relieves nasal dryness

If you're interested in reading more about nasal cleansing, refer to the informative book *Neti: Healing Secrets of Yoga and Ayurveda,* by David Frawley (Lotus Press, 2005).

My Favorite Pot

While many companies offer nasal-cleansing pots, the only one that I use and recommend (because it's the best) is the *Ancient Secrets Nasal Cleansing Pot* by Lotus Brands, Inc. It's crafted from sturdy, lead-free ceramic (not plastic) and coated with food-grade sealant glaze. It features heavy-duty construction and is dishwasher safe. This pot makes nasal irrigation easy and enjoyable. For more information on nasal cleansing and this product, visit: **www.SusanSmithJones.com** and click on *Susan's Favorite Products*. It's available in many better natural-food stores and herb shops. To order it directly, visit: **www.ancient-secrets.com/neti.cfm**, or call: (877) 263-9456.

✳ ✻ ✳

THE HEALING POWER OF SLEEP

"What lies behind us, and what lies before us, are tiny matters compared to what lies within us."

— RALPH WALDO EMERSON

Over the past 40 years, Americans have cut their snooze time by one to two hours per night. We now sleep less than people in any other industrialized country. Chronic sleeping problems afflict as many as 70 million Americans, costing the nation billions in medical expenses, accidents, and lost productivity, according to a new study. Last year, doctors wrote a record 43 million prescriptions for sleeping pills. What's going on? How does this deprivation affect our bodies?

There's nothing more physically restorative than good sleep, and plenty of it, night after night after night. Lack in this area affects everything—job performance, schoolwork, health, and family harmony. Women, especially mothers, are the most deprived, losing about nine hours of sleep each week. Sleep debt impacts relationships, too. According to a very recent National Sleep Foundation poll, 25 percent of couples say they're too tired for sex. And it's been shown that if you only get six hours of sleep nightly, your mental functioning will be on about the same level as that of a drunk driver.

Lack of sleep also undermines your body's ability to deal with stress. One way to tell if you're getting enough shut-eye is to see if you wake at a regular time without an alarm. If you require a buzzer to get out of bed in the morning, you're not getting enough sleep.

How much do you need each day? As I mentioned in Part I, adults need 8¼ hours of sleep nightly to maximize their ability to function daily. Adolescents require 9¼ hours; preschoolers have to get 12 hours; toddlers need 13 hours; and babies need 14–18 hours.

Too Tired to Lose Weight

As I mentioned earlier in this book, researchers now are discovering that sleep affects the hormones that regulate satiety, hunger, and how efficiently you burn calories. Put simply, too little sleep makes you hungry, especially for those foods that are high in calories and low in nutritional value. These include processed junk foods, especially those made with white sugar and flour, and fried items such as French fries and potato chips. Lack of sleep also primes your body to hold on to the calories you eat.

Are you interested in slimming down? If so, more sleep may provide some help. Researchers at Columbia University in New York City found that people who slept six hours a night were 23 percent more likely to be obese than those who slept between seven and nine hours. Folks who snoozed for five hours were 50 percent more likely to be obese, and those who slept four hours or less were 73 percent more likely. So if you're eager to drop a few pounds, make getting ample sleep each night a permanent habit in your lifestyle.

In my private practice, as well as in my holistic-health seminars around the country, I recommend quality sleep because it makes for better relationships. People sometimes think of ennui as being a natural part of relationships, but with enough sleep, conjugal happiness can last. If everyone would just get more sleep and feel more rested, people would be more thoughtful toward one another, and family dynamics would run more smoothly. We'd all be happier and in better moods—adults and children. What a wonderful gift that would be for families, friends, business associates, and communities.

Too Tired to Drive

A few of the reasons people sleep less now than they did a century ago are electric lighting; the shift to an urban, industrialized economy; and the debilitating habit of watching late-night television. The result of this sleep deprivation has been a disruption of basic body metabolism. With workloads and daily stress increasing for many Americans, these issues loom larger than ever for both individuals and society.

Consistent lack of sleep can lead to a variety of health problems, including toxic buildup, premature aging, weight gain, depression, irritability, impatience, low sex drive, memory loss, lethargy, relationship problems, and accidents—and at least 1,500 reported "drowsy driving" fatalities each year. The instant you feel sleepy at the wheel of an automobile—when your eyelids get heavy—get off the road. Cars are so cozy and comfortable these days that it's easy to forget that when you're driving, you're engaging in a very dangerous activity.

Sleepy people are dangerous to themselves and others. The National Highway Traffic Safety Administration estimates that sleep deprivation plays a role in nearly 100,000 traffic accidents each year; it also has been cited as a leading cause of workplace mishaps and has contributed to such disasters as the Chernobyl nuclear-reactor meltdown and the *Exxon Valdez* spill.

Too Tired to Think Straight

Karine Spiegel and colleagues at the University of Chicago asked research participants to stay in bed just 4 hours per night for six nights, then 12 hours per night for the next seven nights. When subjects were sleep deprived, their blood sugars, cortisol, and sympathetic-nervous-system activity rose, and their thyrotropin (a hormone that regulates thyroid function) level fell. In other words, the results of this study show that chronic sleep deprivation forces the body into a fight-or-flight response, pushing blood sugars and other hormone-related functions out of kilter.

Among other things, higher cortisol levels lead to memory loss, an increase in fat storage, and a decrease in muscle (the perfect combination if you want to seem stupid and gain weight). But if you'd like to increase muscle mass—which is necessary to create a fit, lean body—you need at least eight hours of sound sleep nightly to encourage muscle maintenance and growth and the release of human growth hormone, which helps keep you youthful and strong. In other words, sufficient sleep can help make you slimmer.

Lack of shut-eye can also accelerate the aging process. Spiegel found that participants who only slept four hours a night for one week metabolized glucose 40 percent more slowly than usual, which is similar to the rate seen in elderly people. Glucose metabolism quickly returned to normal after the participants got a full night's sleep every night for a week.

How do you know if you're sleep deprived? If you become sluggish, drowsy, or fatigued, particularly after lunch or in the middle of the afternoon, you fall into this category. If you have difficulty getting up in the morning—one of my clients often slumbers on through two alarms—you're also in this group.

A staggering 95 percent of Americans suffer from a sleep disorder at some time in their lives, and 60 percent suffer from a persistent one, according to William C. Dement, M.D., Ph.D., author of *The Promise of Sleep.* When it comes to sleep, researchers and other experts say that *most people require a minimum of eight hours nightly.* Every hour you lose adds to your sleep indebtedness, and you can't expect to catch up by sleeping late one day a week. The loss accumulates progressively and contributes to long-term health problems. And this problem isn't limited to adults—as I've already mentioned, children and teens actually need even more than grown-ups. Sleep loss affects how they learn and increases the chance of accidents, depression, and violent or aggressive behavior.

Nap Time

Recognizing that many of us simply can't get to bed any earlier or wake up any later, a few enlightened businesses are adopting the pioneering view that napping actually can promote productivity. Some companies even provide special nap rooms for employees. Naps should be recognized as a powerful tool in battling fatigue.

However, if you have insomnia, naps actually can aggravate your night's sleep. By taking the edge off your sleepiness, an afternoon snooze may make it even harder for you to drift off at night. In other words, if you're drowsy because of insomnia, napping should be *avoided.*

Naps are also *not* recommended after meals. It's natural to want to lie down after eating because distension of the stomach increases the deep-sleep drive. The problem is that if you overeat, the digestive process may interfere with the *quality* of your rest; and conversely, sleep may interfere with processing your food. You're better off to allow digestion to occur *before* sleeping because these functions tend to work better when performed separately.

Inducing Good Sleep

So far, we've explored how lack of sleep can lead to a variety of health problems, including weight gain, accelerated aging, depression, irritability, impatience, low sex drive, memory loss, lethargy, relationship problems, accidents, and toxic buildup. In this final section, we'll focus on tips for better sleep.

Increasing evening body heat is a very effective way to promote deeper sleep. Normally, your temperature hits a peak two hours before bedtime. Then, as it declines, melatonin is released, and your body gets physiologically ready for sleep. The bigger the drop in temperature, the deeper the descent into sleep. People with insomnia don't have the normal reduction in temperature, so they aren't as ready for deep sleep.

Heating up with exercise four hours before bedtime (to allow enough time for the adrenaline release caused by exertion to wear off) can assist the physiological drive into deep sleep. A hot bath two hours before bedtime or a sauna early in the evening can be good alternatives. This overall increase in body temperature, with its accompanying big drop back to normal, helps promote sound, deep sleep. A cool room and pillow also can be helpful. Place a zip-top bag filled with ice on top of your pillowcase and remove it when you go to bed.

Another way to assure more quality shut-eye is to make sure the bed is for sleep and sex only; avoid working, eating, or watching TV in bed. Natural fiber (as opposed to synthetic) sheets and pajamas (if you wear any) promote sound sleep. Reading until you drift off is okay, but stick to inspirational, uplifting, or calming works, such as my books and audio programs *Be Healthy~Stay Balanced: 21 Simple Choices to Create More Joy & Less Stress, Choose to Live Peacefully, Choose to Live Fully, Wired to Meditate,* and *EveryDay Health—Pure & Simple.*

The ideal bedroom is dark and quiet with plenty of fresh air. Consider adding green plants to your decor—their extra oxygen helps you rest well. I also find that two or three drops of pure essential lavender oil on my pillowcase help me relax.

A good mattress and a few extra pillows are essential. How firm they should be is a personal choice, but if they're uneven and worn out, they should be replaced as soon as possible. I don't recommend using the same mattress for more than ten years. When sleeping on your side, place a pillow between your legs; on your back, put it under your knees. Avoid sleeping on your front (stomach) as this can lead to severe lower-back pain and wrinkles on your face.

Don't eat too close to bedtime—a big, spicy meal may cause sleep-inhibiting indigestion. Choose your evening meals wisely. Carbohydrate-rich foods help send the amino acid tryptophan to the brain, which may induce sleep. Proteins inhibit this chemical's journey, making you more alert. So if you're really hungry after dinner, choose a healthful carb snack. Note that alcohol blocks the restful sleep experienced during the REM cycle. Get a balance of minerals throughout the day—especially calcium, magnesium, and iron—because these have a sedative effect; deficiencies may keep you awake. This book (as well as *The Healing Power of NatureFoods* and *Be Healthy~Stay Balanced*) identifies specific foods that will help you sleep better, have more energy, and look years younger than your age.

Sweet Dreams

As I mentioned previously, there's nothing more restorative for the body than plenty of good sleep on a regular basis. So if you want to be the best you can be, make this a nonnegotiable habit because it will have a positive impact on every area—body, mind, emotions, and spirit. With enough shut-eye, you'll heal your physical self, feel more empowered, have more confidence, and know that you can face whatever comes each day with aplomb and élan.

If everyone would just get more sleep and feel more rested, we'd be kinder toward one another; and family, friend, and business relationships would run more smoothly. Sweet, delicious sleep is a wonderful gift to give to yourself—and to others! (For more encouraging information on sleep, please visit: **www.PagingSusan.com**.)

❈ ❊ ❈

THE HEALING POWER
OF A HEALTHY METABOLISM

*"It is, by far, much easier to preserve health
than to regain it."*

— BENJAMIN FRANKLIN

While millions are starving to death around the world, Americans have the dubious honor of being the fattest people on the globe (and 50 percent of us are obese). Is it any wonder that we're preoccupied with our waistlines? U.S. residents spend more than $40 billion a year on diet foods, programs, and pills and other "guaranteed" weight-loss regimens and products. Yet, according to the National Center of Health Statistics, we're getting fatter all the time.

Experts call obesity an American epidemic—one that brings with it major health problems. Heart disease, endometrial (uterine) and possibly breast cancer, high cholesterol, high blood pressure, immune dysfunction, osteoarthritis, stroke, gout, sleep disorders, gallstones, and diabetes all are associated with obesity. Put in a more positive way, *losing even a little weight may improve your health and well-being significantly—and prevent those very same diseases.*

Undereating is also a problem, and disorders such as anorexia and bulimia are on the rise. Advertising for women's clothing contributes to the problem by using models who look like waifs. Consider Barbie, a doll that's part of most little girls' upbringing. This model of good looks and the perfect body is giving the wrong message about what a healthy woman should look like. Were Barbie an actual person, her body fat would be so low that she probably wouldn't even be able to menstruate. As little girls treasure the doll and teens try to emulate her, she has one accessory that's consistently missing—food.

Surveys indicate that most people are unhappy with their weight or the shape of their bodies. Currently, half of the women and a quarter of the men in the United States are trying to lose weight and reshape themselves. The sad thing is that the majority are going about it in the wrong way, the hard way—by dieting, which doesn't work! Throw away books that tell you that you can lose weight and keep it off without moving a muscle. They're rip-offs. Dieting isn't the cure for excess fat. After you finish such a program, you may have lost some fat, but *you haven't lost your tendency to get fat.*

The control mechanism for obesity isn't diet; it's muscle metabolism. Your basal metabolic rate is the speed at which your body utilizes energy. Put another way, it has to do with how efficiently you burn calories, the measuring unit of heat energy. When metabolism is higher, you burn more fat and have an easier time losing pounds (fat) and maintaining your ideal body weight. You can feed yourself the best food and vitamin supplements in the world, but if the muscles aren't tuned up—if they're not exercised—they won't burn up the calories. As you age, if you don't continue to keep your muscles exercised, your metabolism will slow down, and you'll gain weight more easily than you did when you were younger. *Exercise is the key to controlling metabolism.*

Two out of three people who go on a diet will regain their weight in one year or less; 97 percent will gain it back within five years. In fact, a majority of dieters who lose weight will eventually end up with even more fat than they had before they started the regimen. To make matters worse, these people typically lose lean body mass or muscle, which is the last thing you want to do.

If you're overweight, you need to retrain your body so that it burns up *all* of the calories it gets, storing none as fat. Yes, you may need a diet at the start to help break bad eating habits, retrain your taste buds, jump-start your metabolism, and lose some excess pounds. But long-term weight control requires a change in body chemistry so that you won't get heavy all over again. And *exercise* is the only way to change your metabolism so that you convert fewer calories to fat. You need aerobic exercise to burn the fat and weight lifting to build up your muscles, which, in turn, increases metabolism.

8 Steps to Accelerate Fat Loss & Create a Healthy, Fit Body for Life

Here are some tips for increasing your metabolism, selecting the right exercise and foods, and making good choices to create a fit, healthy body.

1. Increase your muscle mass. Muscle burns fat—it's that simple. Exercise increases muscle, tones it, alters its chemistry, and increases your metabolic rate. When you work out regularly, you actually burn calories even when you're sleeping, but you must exercise correctly to get the best results. Before I describe the best methods to lose fat and increase metabolism, let's briefly explore why lean muscle tissue is so important.

More muscle means a faster metabolism because it uses more energy to exist. It's a highly metabolic tissue, burning five times as many calories as most other body tissues, pound for pound. In other words, it requires more oxygen and calories to sustain itself. When you have more muscle mass, you burn more calories than someone less muscular, even when you're both sitting still. That's why people who build muscle have an easier time maintaining a healthful weight. They're simply more efficient at burning calories.

If you increase muscle mass, you raise the number of calories your body is using every moment—not just during exercise, but also at work, at play, and even when sleeping. The addition of ten pounds of muscle will burn approximately 500 extra calories per day. You'd have to jog five miles a day, seven days a week, to achieve that without the alteration in body composition. Ten extra pounds of muscle can burn a pound of fat in one week—that's 52 pounds of fat a year!

To increase muscle, you must engage in weight lifting, also known as strength or resistance training. Actually it's not the lifting itself, but the physiological effects that take place in the 48 hours *afterward,* during the recovery period that enhance metabolism. In other words, very little fat is burned during the strength-training sessions; but *lots* of it melts down over the next couple of days.

Long after you've finished lifting, your fat-burning enzymes are working harder than ever to repair the damage. They must replace the sugar that was used by the sugar-burning enzymes, and to build up the supplies, your body burns fat. It takes a lot of energy to restore sugar (glycogen is stored muscle sugar that's used up during weight lifting), which means that lots of calories are burned. *All* of this energy must be supplied by the fat-burning enzymes. That's why you must make this type of exercise a part of your fat-loss/vitality program—*it stimulates metabolism and fat burning.*

I can't emphasize this enough: The best way to increase lean muscle mass is through resistance training, which means weight lifting or resistance machines—barbells, dumbbells, machines, cables, or even "free-hand" movements such as push-ups, sit-ups (crunches), and dips. All it takes to add ten pounds of muscle is a regular weight-training program involving 30–40 minutes, three times a week, for about six months.

2. Increase your aerobic exercise. This trains muscles to burn fat and increase metabolism, and it means exercising with oxygen, not being winded or out of breath. These types of exercises, which are nonstop and fairly gentle, change your metabolism. Here's a key point to keep in mind: *Muscles burn fat only in the presence of oxygen.* For example, if you're jogging with your husband and he's breezing along and singing a song, while you're so out of breath that you can barely put two syllables together, he's reducing fat, but your fat-burning mechanisms have shut down. Muscles consume two kinds of fuel—sugar (glucose) and fat. Your lean tissues really do prefer to burn fat because it's more efficient; there's more of it, so it lasts a long time and produces lots of energy.

Does that mean you shouldn't do high-intensity sprints every so often? No, as I'll explain shortly, but you must make aerobic exercise part of your fitness program at least five days a week if you want to lose fat and tone up. By using the big muscles of the thighs and buttocks in an activity that's steady and nonstop (such as cross-country skiing, bicycling, rowing, walking, and hiking), which makes you inhale deeply but doesn't leave you out of breath, you're supplying oxygen to the muscles, which promotes fat burning and makes you use up more food calories.

3. Add higher intensity bursts to your exercise plan. I work some high-intensity activities into my exercise program a few times each week. For example, if I'm hiking, I'll increase my pace up a hill for 30–90 seconds every so often. (Notice I didn't say "a breakneck run"; just go a little faster than usual.) If you're cycling, pedal faster for several seconds. High-intensity bursts of exercise help burn fat. Why? When you force your body to raise the level of exertion for a short burst of "getting winded," you're making yourself recover under stress (in other words, while you continue to exercise). This little sprint adds intensity without causing injury. And those fat-burning enzymes are realizing that not only do they need to grow when you're doing regular aerobic activity, but now they must increase even faster. In other words, *a few moments of exercising just a little bit harder than usual will help force you to recover while still exercising, which will* *burn more fat.* If you're just a beginner and have never worked out before, wait for about one month before adding in these bursts, and then pump it up if your doctor says you can.

4. Graze. Liquid meals, diet pills, and special packaged foods aren't your answer to increasing metabolism, weight control, or better health. Instead, and in addition to regular exercise, learn how to eat so that your body becomes an efficient fat-burning machine.

The results of four national surveys show that most people try to lose weight by eating 1,000–1,500 calories per day. However, cutting calories to less than 1,200 (if you're a woman) or 1,400 (if you're a man) doesn't provide enough food to be satisfying in the long term. Eating less than these amounts slows down metabolism and makes it difficult to get adequate amounts of certain nutrients, such as folic acid, magnesium, and zinc.

The typical dieter will often skip meals. And as research points out, the worst one to drop, if you want to increase your metabolism, is breakfast. This temporary fasting state sends a signal to the body that food is scarce. As a result, the stress hormones (including cortisol) increase, and the body begins "lightening the load" and shedding its muscle tissue, which decreases the need for food. By the next feeding, the pancreas is sensitized and will sharply increase blood insulin levels, which is the body's signal to make fat. And if you're insulin-resistant, as many sedentary people are, you make extra amounts of this hormone (insulin) and create/deposit fat very easily, especially if you eat refined carbohydrates. Have you ever wondered how sumo wrestlers get so big? They fast and then gorge themselves. Clearly, this approach is absolutely counterproductive if your goal is to lose fat.

If you want to increase your metabolism, it's best to eat several small healthful meals each day, about every three hours or so (five to six meals daily). This "grazing" approach keeps your metabolism stoked. It also keeps you from feeling deprived—a chief complaint of anyone who has ever been on a diet. If you want to know the specific foods to eat to accelerate fat loss and create a healthy, fit body, please refer to this book and *The Healing Power of NatureFoods.* You also may want to check out my books *Recipes for Health Bliss: Using NatureFoods to Rejuvenate Your Body & Life* (available from Hay House, June 2009) and *Be Healthy~Stay Balanced.*

5. Drink at least two quarts of water each day. Water is very important in helping maintain a healthy metabolic rate and a fit body. It's essential to drink at least two quarts of water per day (at least eight glasses) between meals, more if you're physically active. This suppresses your appetite naturally. Have a large glass about 15–20 minutes before each meal or snack. I cannot stress enough how simply drinking purified water contributes greatly to fat loss and the reshaping of your body, even if you don't change any of your other habits.

The liver's main functions are detoxification and regulation of metabolism. The kidneys also can get rid of toxins if they have sufficient water. Drinking enough water daily allows the kidneys to spare the liver some of its purifying efforts, which allows it to metabolize more fat. Adequate water also will decrease bloating and edema caused by fluid accumulation by flushing out sodium, acidic wastes, and other toxins.

6. **Eat good fats.** Sedentary, overweight people tend to eat a higher-fat diet than those of healthful weight. Fatty foods slow metabolism, which causes the body to convert dietary fat into body fat very easily. Gram for gram, fats not only have more than twice the calories of carbohydrates and proteins (nine compared to four), they also burn only 2 percent of their calories in the process of being stored as fat. By contrast, protein and carbohydrates burn about 25 percent of their calories during the same process.

It's considerably more difficult to convert protein and carbohydrates into body fat because you actually burn calories doing so. If you currently are maintaining your weight on 3,000 calories per day, and then decrease the fat from 40 percent to 20 percent, you can lose one pound of fat in about three weeks—while at the same time eating 20 percent more food from complex carbohydrates and protein. The bottom line is this: *Eating too much fat (especially from animal products) makes you fat.*

But not all fats make this happen. In fact, you can also fight fat with healthful fat. Sounds paradoxical, doesn't it? Omega-3 fatty acids actually can help increase your metabolic rate. They also rid the body of excess fluids and can increase your energy level. Omega-6 (LA) fatty acids (especially gamma linolenic acid or GLA) also are essential to a healthy metabolism and are less likely to be deficient in a healthful diet. Good sources of omega-3 fatty acids include flaxseed, flax meal, flax oil, walnuts, organic hemp milk, nuts, and leafy green vegetables. For family or friends who still consume animal products, omega-3s are also available in certain fish, such as salmon.

7. **Meditate to reduce stress.** Sometimes the things that you experience can put a burden on you physically by causing endocrine or hormonal events that

stress your body. Medical experts now believe that these stresses are at the root of many degenerative disease processes. In other words, stress has a biological as well as an emotional effect on you, and it can diminish your body's ability to fortify, protect, regenerate, and heal itself over time.

Stress can be triggered by emotions, such as anger, fear, worry, grief, and guilt. It may be the result of an injury or trauma, an accident, or surgery. Everyday pressures like family squabbles, impossible bosses, unfaithful spouses, unruly teens, and overdue bills can cause strain, as can an extreme change in sleep pattern, diet, exercise, and even climate. So can chronic illness, pain, allergies, and inflammation. Too much work—too much of almost anything—can create tension.

Produced by the adrenal glands and commonly known as the "stress hormone," cortisol helps the body cope with all types of stress, from infection to fright, from a major job change or relocation to divorce or the death of a loved one. Whether you're facing an emergency, an accident, a confrontation, or just doing your job or getting some exercise, cortisol is there to get you up and going and through the day. It floods your system to assist you in emergencies and helps provide nutrients you need to cope with stress. Normally, once you've managed the stressful circumstances, the brain shuts off the production of cortisol, your physical reactions subside, and you quickly return to normal.

But there's another side of the story. If the brain perceives that stress is ongoing or chronic, it can override the messages to shut off cortisol production. Creation of the hormone then stays elevated because the brain thinks the body needs it to cope with what's going on. So as important and necessary as cortisol is, you can have too much of it. If too great an amount stays in your body for too long, a damaging cycle can begin that can lead to blood-sugar problems, fat accumulation, compromised immune function, exhaustion, bone loss, and even heart disease. If you experience one major stress after another, and if you haven't created ways to reduce and release that tension, it can have a detrimental effect on your waistline and your health.

A daily practice of meditation has been shown to cause a generalized reduction in numerous physiological and biochemical stress indicators—such as decreases in heart rate, respiration rate, stress hormones, and pulse—and an increase in oxygen consumption and slow alpha waves, brain waves associated with relaxation. Meditation is being used successfully by people suffering from chronic pain and conditions such as cancer and heart disease, as well as stress-related disorders such as abdominal pain, chronic diarrhea, and ulcers.

For more than 35 years, I've been an avid meditator; and I give workshops and seminars on the benefits of this practice, offering simple ways to make it part of your lifestyle. If you want to learn more about its salutary effects on body, mind, emotions, and spirit or find out how to do it, please refer to my books-on-tape *Wired to Meditate* and *Choose to Live Peacefully,* which are available on my Websites: **www.PagingSusan.com** and **www.SusanSmithJones.com** or by calling: (800) 843-5743, Monday through Friday, 9 A.M. to 4 P.M. PT.

8. **Nourish your spirit.** This is necessary in order to maintain a healthy body. The real epidemic in our society is spiritual heart disease—the experience of low self-esteem combined with feelings of loneliness, isolation, and alienation that pervade our culture. I write and talk about this in detail in my books and audio programs *Choose to Live Peacefully,* Be Healthy~Stay Balanced, and EveryDay Health—*Pure & Simple.* Many people who suffer from spiritual malaise use food or stimulants such as drugs, caffeine, alcohol, sex, gambling, or overwork (or almost anything to the extreme) to numb the pain and get through the day.

Stretching, deep breathing, and meditation will relax your mind, and you'll experience a greater sense of peace and well-being. From there, you'll be able to make eating and exercise decisions—and other lifestyle choices—that are life-enhancing rather than self-destructive. Engage in physical activities that nourish your body and soul. Cherished activities of mine include hiking, in-line skating, gardening, walking in a botanical or flower garden, stretching, and yoga.

In conclusion, dieting alone isn't sufficient to achieve healthful, permanent weight loss; good nutrition combined with regular aerobic exercise is better. But a program that includes strength training, aerobic exercise, sensible eating, stress management, meditation, and other nourishment for your spirit provides an unbeatable combination for reaching and maintaining your ideal weight; improving your metabolism; creating a fit, lean body; and celebrating life.

THE HEALING POWER OF BEAUTIFUL SKIN

"'Hope' is the thing with feathers—
That perches in the soul . . ."

— EMILY DICKINSON

The skin is the largest single organ of the body and comes in many colors, textures, and patterns. Imagine a material that's waterproof, yet can let out water and oil; that can protect like a suit of armor, and yet is infinitely sensitive to touch; that remains strong yet penetrably flexible. It's also a beautiful material— whether pink, brown, yellow, black, or any of the many shades in between.

It's amazing to think that all we ever see of one another—and the basis of so many of our judgments about each other—is skin surfaces. This substance is continually growing from within, creating new cells that push their way outward. The skin on the palms of our hands renews every 24 hours, our faces every 7 days, and on the rest of our body every 30 days. Yet the skin, perhaps more than any other part of us, tells the world how we feel mentally and physically as well as how we care for and respect our bodies. American Indians used to diagnose body ailments by the lines in the face.

The skin of an adult covers a surface area of about 18–21 square feet. Weighing in at about six pounds, the skin is about one-eighth of an inch thick, varying at different areas of the body. It's well supplied with a variety of glands, blood vessels, and nerves and consists of three distinct layers: the epidermis (which is composed of four sub-layers), the dermis, and the subcutaneous fat. The dermis layer relies on the protein collagen to keep it in mint condition by acting as a supporter and as a major building block of the skin. Elastin, another protein, gives the organ its supple, elastic quality.

In an average square inch of skin, there are approximately 200 blood and lymph vessels, 100 oil glands, 650 sweat glands, 28 motor nerves, 13 sense receptors for cold, 78 sense receptors for heat, 1,300 tactile receptors, and 65 hairs, plus millions of independent cell forms.

Functions of the Skin

Two million pores cover the body's surface and function together as an efficient cooling system. Exercise can raise internal temperature up to seven degrees above normal, and the body dissipates that excess heat through perspiration, which evaporates on the skin. Besides cooling and protecting the body, the skin also serves as a sense organ. It's thought that a fetus probably receives most sensations through the skin; and from the moment of birth, humans require touching and physical affection just as much as food. The skin is an organ of amazing complexity that we're only beginning to understand, and remarkably, no two people on earth have identical skin formation—not even twins—just as each of us has unique fingerprints.

The sun is the body's most effective, efficient, and least expensive source of vitamin D, appropriately termed the "sunshine" vitamin. The action of the ultraviolet rays activates a form of cholesterol that's present in the skin, converting it to vitamin D. Most of the body's needs for this nutrient can be met from monitored exposure to sunlight and eating small amounts of certain foods such as sprouted seeds, mushrooms, and sunflower seeds.

On the other hand, many people still feel that a deep golden tan is the mark of the leisure class, portraying health and beauty. The sun does have some additional beneficial effects, such as helping clear up acne, relaxing tired muscles, and creating positive psychological effects; but too much of this good thing is just about the skin's worst enemy.

Beautifying Your Skin with 8 Easy Steps

Besides using common sense when it comes to sun exposure, refer to the following proven tips to help revitalize your skin.

1. Exercise: This improves circulation throughout the body and creates an increase in body heat. The elevated temperature draws blood into the skin surface, increasing dermal capillary circulation; and with greater blood flow comes more nourishment and a better complexion. Your skin benefits from most types of heat: saunas, exercise, aromatherapeutic baths, and massage.

2. Sleep: This is not only good for overall health, but is imperative for healthy skin. Like so many other organs, it regenerates and heals most effectively while you sleep, so getting adequate rest will help keep your skin healthy and beautiful.

3. Diet: A healthful diet is essential for healthy skin. Nutrients in plant foods nourish the skin and provide all of the elements necessary to keep skin looking youthful. Not only do these colorful, fiber-rich foods help keep the digestive system moving smoothly, but they're also rich in antioxidants like vitamins C and E, various carotenoids, and flavonoids that are beneficial to the skin. Eating an antioxidant-rich diet also bolsters your protection against disease.

4. Water: This is as important as diet for keeping your skin healthy. In fact, you'll see a difference in appearance in just three days if you drink at least a half gallon (64 ounces) of purified water every day. I usually drink at least 80 ounces daily, and even more on days when I work out for more than two hours. Increased water consumption will make your skin softer, smoother, and more toned. When you fly, take a small spray bottle and spritz your skin every 15 minutes. The mist will refresh your skin and increase the spirit-lifting negative ions around you, so you'll arrive at your destination with a healthy glow and a more positive attitude.

5. Vitamin C: This is one of your skin's best friends. Collagen and elastin, the two building blocks of this organ, are only made by the fibroblast cells with the use of vitamin C. Sags, bags, droops, puckers, blotches, and spider veins can be signs of vitamin-C deficiency. You can apply this nutrient directly to your skin in the form of lotions, creams, serums, and oils (see "Skin-care products," item 7 in this list); and it also should be ingested. A stress-filled life increases your need. Excellent food sources include oranges, strawberries, kiwi, tomatoes, grapefruit, dark green leafy vegetables, broccoli, broccoli sprouts, bell peppers, and papaya.

6. Positive attitude and meditation: These two elements bring vitality to your life by reducing stress, anxiety, and pain. Scientists are even discovering that meditation helps keep you wrinkle free and healthy; those who engage in this practice regularly look 12–15 years younger than nonmeditators of the same age. Meditation also reduces tension in the body and helps foster a positive attitude.

7. Skin-care products: One of the most frequent comments I receive, whether participating in media talk shows, giving workshops, or consulting with clients, is this: "Susan, your skin looks so healthy and youthful. What skin products do you use?" I usually respond by saying that healthy skin starts on the inside by eating a top-quality diet (as described in this book) and drinking plenty of water each day. Of course, you must get enough sleep, keep stress to a minimum, protect yourself from excessive sun exposure, exercise regularly, dry skin brush daily, and cultivate a positive attitude.

It's also important to use good skin-care products. For more than 30 years, most of what I've used on my skin has been made by the eminent company *Reviva Labs.* Established in 1973, Reviva realized long before it was in vogue that *natural* ingredients were essential in order to make truly healthful skin products. While the brand offers a complete line of superb products for all skin types, four of my favorites include their *Light Skin Peel, Green Papaya Hydrogen Peroxide Facial Mask, Almond and Carrot Oil Mask,* and *Optimum Antioxidant Facial Mask with Artichoke.*

Once a week, I use the Light Skin Peel on my face, neck, and the backs of my hands. A nonchemical peel, this celebrated product helps improve color tone, refine and smooth texture, and brighten skin surface. The beautiful feel and look of your complexion after the peel is removed is the result of its combination of ingredients—papaya extract, salicylic acid, almond and root extracts, zinc oxide, and kaolin—that dissolve dead skin and leave you with a very healthy glow.

Then, usually right after the peel, but sometimes on an alternate day, I follow up with the Green Papaya Hydrogen Peroxide Facial Mask. Beyond cleansing pores of impurities and pollutants, it delivers fresh ingredients that will help your skin look clearer and more radiant. Because of the high percentage of green papaya, you'll also benefit from a mild exfoliation without redness or irritation. This is a soothing, soft, nonhardening, nondrying mask that can benefit any skin type—even sensitive skin like mine; it will leave your skin sparkling clean, smooth, and glowing. I use it on my face, neck, décolleté, and the backs of my hands. (For more information on Reviva's Optimum Antioxidant Facial Mask with Artichoke, see the earlier section on Artichokes.)

You can find these items, and most of the Reviva product line, at better natural-food stores. You also can order these products through the Reviva Website: **http://www.revivalabs.com** or by calling: (800) 257-7774.

8. Dry skin brushing: This is one of the best ways to create beautiful skin all over your body. It has been popular in Europe for decades and is finally beginning to catch on here in America. Not only does it improve the appearance of your skin, giving you a healthy glow, but it also helps your body eliminate toxins. Because dry skin brushing is not well known here, I've included a section that describes everything you need to know about this beneficial practice.

The Healing Power of Dry Skin Brushing

If you haven't yet tried skin brushing, you're in for a treat! As author Shazzie writes in her enlightening book *Detox Your World,* you can stimulate and cleanse your lymphatic system by using a dry vegetable brush. Some people follow the traditional Chinese method and use a loofah (sponge) to brush the skin, but I feel that approach is too harsh and not as effective as using bristles.

The skin is the largest organ in the body, and a quarter of your daily elimination comes through it. Your lymph nodes play a role in this process by filtering and holding toxic materials. Some health advocates think that stimulating the nodes with skin brushing helps them detoxify and release these harmful materials faster. When you skin brush, you not only help your lymph system clean itself, you also keep your pores open, encouraging your body to discharge other toxins and metabolic waste. Products such as deodorants, soaps, and lotions, as well as synthetic clothing, all can play a part in causing more toxins to enter via your skin. Skin brushing can coax them out.

If you do this for just three days in a row, you'll start to notice your skin texture become smoother, your color might change and lose any gray tinge, and your body will tone up so cellulite is less visible. Here are some more of the many benefits of skin brushing:

* Skin becomes tighter.
* Dead, clogged skin is removed.
* Cellulite is reduced.
* Digestion improves.
* Cells are renewed at a faster rate.
* Your lymph is cleansed.
* Your immune system is strengthened.
* Your whole body is stimulated, so it works more efficiently.

How to Brush Your Skin

This is quite a simple technique for something so valuable. Simply brush your skin once each day while you're waiting for your bath to run or shower to warm up. When engaging in a detoxifying program, you might benefit from doing it twice daily. It will take you only two to five minutes to brush your skin.

Go into a warm room, remove all of your clothes, and make sure your body is dry. You can use circular motions or stroke in one direction, toward the heart. I generally brush in this order: soles of feet, ankles, calves, thighs, tummy, buttocks, hands, arms, back, and chest. When working on your stomach, brush from the upper left, then down and around in a circular motion. Imagine that you are following your colon. You can use a smaller and much softer brush on your face, or you can omit it.

Once you've brushed yourself all over, you can repeat it once or twice more if you want, or you can go and enjoy your bath or shower. If you can bear it, have a cool rinse after you bathe, as this will help your blood circulation. After a few days, you'll automatically be less tentative as your skin becomes used to the brush.

As most household dust comes from the skin we shed, you can imagine how your brush may end up! It will last for years and stay beautiful, however, if you wash it in mild soap or shampoo every week or two and let it dry naturally. I use a mild tea-tree-oil liquid soap.

Invest in the Best Dry Skin Brush

Look for a dry brush at your local natural-food store or bath- and beauty-supply store. Make sure it has natural bristles (as opposed to nylon or another synthetic material) and a long handle so you can reach all those hard-to-get-to places on your body.

My favorite dry skin brush—the one I use and recommend in all of my work—can be ordered through the contact information that follows. There's one brush for your body and another special brush to use on your face; you'll want to get both of them. Also, to keep your skin glowing and your body vibrantly healthy and rejuvenated, I encourage you to undertake four detoxification programs each year, concomitant with dry skin brushing. I do this for 7 to 10 days with each change of season. My favorite complete detox program—which I highly recommend because of its efficacy—is called the *Internal Cleanse Tool Kit*. It provides everything you need to embark on a cleansing program in your own home; you don't even need to take time off work. This dynamic process will help you look and feel your very best year-round. Who doesn't want that?

When I undertake a quarterly detox program, I also take extra capsules of a superlative, 100 percent organic, whole-foods supplement called *Super Organic Rainbow Salad*. It's a one-of-a-kind, "full color spectrum" nutritional supplement (in capsule form) that combines a variety of superfoods—everything your body needs to take your health to the highest level. You'll want to take a few capsules daily, and then take extra capsules during the days you're on a detox program.

For more information on these products or to order, please visit: **www.bernardjensen.org** or call: (888) 743-1790 or (760) 471-9977 (outside the United States).

Take charge of your health today by following all the suggestions in this section. Dry skin brushing is a good place to start, and you'll see a difference in only three days. I wish you radiant health and youthful vitality.

❋ ❋ ❋

THE HEALING POWER
OF SWEATING & SAUNAS

"You see things and say 'Why?'
But I dream things that never were
and say 'Why not?'"

— GEORGE BERNARD SHAW

Saunas, in one form or another, have been used across ages and oceans. Cultures around the world have recognized the relaxing benefits of rendered heat within a warm, welcoming space. From the elaborate bath/sauna/exercise complexes of the Romans to the Japanese to the simple but effective "sweat lodge" structures of the Scandinavians and Native Americans, heat therapy has been essential for the body to unwind from the stresses and hardships of daily life. These cultures recognized the many therapeutic benefits of the sauna, fully enjoying these benefits in a community setting.

In Finland, the sauna is a historic tradition. According to the late Paavo Airola, in his book *Health Secrets From Europe,* the sauna has been an important part of Finnish life and culture for more than 1,000 years, cherished by every Finnish man, woman, and child. In fact, the custom is credited for much of their rugged vitality and endurance. In a country of approximately five million, there are an estimated 700,000 saunas—one for every seven people! Airola writes, "Most Finnish saunas are in separate buildings specially constructed for this purpose. Every farm has its own sauna, usually built on the shore of a lake or river. Most family houses in the city have saunas built on the lot, usually in the backyard."

Business meetings between strangers in Finland often are conducted in the soothing surroundings of the sauna, and it has been suggested that the combination of high heat and nakedness enabled the Finns to successfully negotiate the international-trade minefields between East and West during the Cold War. There's a saying in Finland that one must behave in the sauna just as in church—it's considered to be very sacred.

What can we learn from the Finns about the benefits of saunas? Sweating is not only an important part of our physical well-being, but in these modern times of water and airborne pollution, toxic chemicals, heavy metals, and poor dietary and exercise habits, the therapeutic internal cleansing of regular sweating is critical to maintain a healthy body and mind.

Dry-Air Saunas vs. Wet Steam Rooms

The hot, dry air of the sauna is therapeutically different from the steam room sauna. The dry atmosphere causes profuse sweating—the air itself absorbing the perspiration. But the water-saturated air of the steam room doesn't readily accept the moisture released by the body. This makes you feel hotter because your sweat doesn't evaporate and carry away the heat. This raises a question: Is it better to be warm on the inside or sweaty on the outside?

That depends on what you want from either system. When exposed to heat of any kind, blood vessels in the skin dilate to allow more blood to flow to the surface. This activates the millions of sweat glands that cover the body. The fluid in the blood hydrates the sweat glands, which pour the water into the skin's surface. As the water evaporates, it draws heat from the body; it's nature's cooling system.

Either the sauna or the steam room can be used to relax and unwind; however, the former clearly has more therapeutic benefits. For one thing, the dry sauna has an advantage because it helps rid the body of more toxic metals picked up from the environment. Of course, the kidneys take out many of these toxins, but a daily sweat can help reduce the accumulation of lead, mercury, and nickel in addition to cadmium, sodium, sulfuric acid, and cholesterol.

The sauna is also more beneficial than the steam room for weight loss because of the different energy expenditures involved in each approach. The sauna places a greater demand on the body in terms of using up calories—therefore assisting in fat loss. The heart has to work harder to send more blood to the capillaries under the skin. The energy required for that process is derived from the conversion of fat and carbohydrates to calories. In addition, the sweat glands must work to produce sweat, thereby expending additional energy (calories). Studies show that a person can burn up to 300 calories during a sauna session, the equivalent of a two to three mile jog or an hour of moderate weight training.

You can lose up to a quart of water (sweating) during a 20-minute sauna. Without replacement, this can lead to disruption of normal heart rhythms and cause fatigue and nausea. Therefore, I recommend drinking fresh fruit juice or water before, during, and after the sauna. Any attempt to lose weight by depriving your body of replacement fluid is extremely risky and can land you in the hospital. Furthermore, I suggest eating plenty of leafy greens and a variety of vegetables and fresh vegetable juices to replace essential minerals such as iron, zinc, copper, and magnesium that are lost in sweat.

Therapeutic Benefits

Sweating caused by overheating the body in a dry sauna also produces these effects:

— It speeds up the metabolic processes of vital organs and inhibits the growth of pathogenic bacteria or viruses. The vital organs and glands, including endocrine and sex glands, are stimulated to increased activity.

— It creates a "fever" reaction that kills potentially dangerous viruses and bacteria and increases the number of leukocytes in the blood, thereby strengthening the immune system—important for fighting colds, flu, and cancer and bolstering resistance to infections. In other words, it increases and accelerates the body's own healing activity and restorative capacity.

— It places demands upon the cardiovascular system, making the heart pump harder and producing a drop in diastolic blood pressure.

— It stimulates vasodilation of peripheral vessels, which relieves pain and speeds healing of sprains, strains, bursitis, peripheral vascular diseases, arthritis, and muscle pain.

— It promotes relaxation, thereby lending a feeling of well-being.

Studies on Artificially Induced Fever

There's a great health benefit of fever. Nobel Prize winner Dr. André Lwoff, a French virologist, believes that high temperature during infection helps combat the growth of virus. "Therefore, fever should not be brought down with drugs," he said. Two medical doctors, Werner Zable and Josef Issels, have this to say about fever: "Artificially induced fever has the greatest potential in the treatment of many diseases, including cancer."

When saunas are used regularly, studies have shown such benefits as improvement of blood circulation, restored youthfulness, toxin and heavy-metal reduction, weight control, cellulite reduction, skin cleansing and rejuvenation, allergy reduction, rash reduction, and muscle- and joint-pain reduction.

With a top-quality infrared sauna, you're able to stay in for a longer time and thus able to reap greater benefits than through the use of other saunas. Also, because your temperature will go up slightly, the body reacts in the normal manner by raising the heart rate to a mild aerobic range, increasing blood flow, widening the capillaries for greater blood flow to sluggish areas, opening up the pores, and creating the deep sweat that flushes out toxins.

On a cautionary note, certain people need to approach saunas slowly and judiciously. Folks over age 60 are in a high-risk group for undiagnosed heart disease. The sauna's no place to find out, so see your doctor before using it. Those who are obese, pregnant, or on regular medication and those who have thyroid, kidney, or respiratory problems; diabetes; or high blood pressure should consult their physicians before using saunas.

Today, sweating is not only "in," it's been proven to be one of the most healthful things a body can do. Nothing beats the feeling and overall well-being or the health benefits you get after you've worked up a good sweat, and the easiest way to a good sweat is to enjoy a sauna.

The Best Sauna

Put bluntly, sitting or lying down on the insalubrious residue of other people's toxic sweat in a public sauna or steam room in a gym (or elsewhere) isn't my idea of a healthy, relaxing experience. Having my own sauna for decades has been a key ingredient of my personal *Be Healthy~Stay Balanced* holistic program. From extensive research on saunas and regular use for more than three decades, my personal preference is the *Thermal Life® Far Infrared Sauna* by High Tech Health. Each top-quality infrared sauna from this company features the best components to help make your sauna experience one of the highlights of your day and the cornerstone of your health program. These include a hypoallergenic design, state-of-the-art Bio-Resonance™ far infrared heaters, two built-in speakers, precision controls, comfortable bench seating, bright lighting for easy reading, built-in fresh air fan, roof vent, window, superb warranty, and so much more. Whether it's a two-, three-, or four-person clinic model, all of these saunas install in 30 minutes (no tools required), warm up in five minutes, and cost only $2 to $4 per month (no plumbing necessary).

For more information or to purchase a sauna, please visit: **www.hightechhealth. com** or call: (800) 794-5355 or (303) 413-8500.

✳ ✺ ✳

THE HEALING POWER OF EXERCISE

"Choose what is best;
habit will soon render it agreeable and easy."

— PYTHAGORAS

Being fit is the key to enjoying life—it will unlock your mental power and physical stamina, as well as give you a positive outlook that will help make each day a celebration. There's nothing that will do more good for you in terms of being vibrantly healthy, energetic, and youthful than a regular fitness program.

Develop a well-rounded regimen that includes strength training, aerobics, and stretching. This triangle will reduce bone loss, maintain strength and muscle mass, keep your energy levels revved, and so much more. Remember these three points: Move, strengthen, and lengthen. When you make your program a top priority in your life and stay committed to it, you'll be well on your way to rejuvenating body, mind, and spirit.

If you need more reasons to exercise, here are 101 I've compiled just for you!

Exercise . . .

1. Increases your self-confidence and self-esteem
2. Improves your digestion
3. Helps you sleep better
4. Gives you more energy
5. Adds sparkle and radiance to your complexion

6. Enhances your immune system

7. Improves your body shape

8. Burns up extra calories

9. Tones and firms your muscles to provide more definition

10. Improves circulation and helps reduce blood pressure

11. Lifts your spirits

12. Reduces tension and quells stress

13. Helps you lose weight and keep it off

14. Builds strength and improves endurance

15. Increases the lean muscle tissue in your body

16. Improves your appetite for healthful foods

17. Alleviates menstrual cramps and mollifies PMS and menopausal symptoms

18. Alters and improves muscle chemistry

19. Increases metabolic rate

20. Enhances coordination and balance

21. Lowers your resting heart rate

22. Increases muscle size through an increase in muscle fibers

23. Improves the storage of glycogen

24. Enables your body to utilize nutrients more efficiently

25. Strengthens your bones

26. Enhances oxygen transport throughout the body

27. Improves liver functioning

28. Increases speed of muscle contraction and therefore reaction time

29. Enhances feedback through the nervous system

30. Strengthens the heart

31. Improves blood flow through the body

32. Increases maximum cardiac output due to an increase in stroke volume

33. Helps release toxins through sweating

34. Increases heart size, strength, and power

35. Improves contractile function of the whole heart

36. Deters heart disease

37. Increases the level of HDL (high-density lipoprotein)

38. Decreases LDL (low-density lipoprotein)

39. Decreases cholesterol and triglycerides

40. Increases total hemoglobin (which carries the red blood cells)

41. Increases alkaline reserve (buffering capacity of the blood)

42. Improves the body's ability to remove lactic acid

43. Improves the body's ability to decrease heart rate after exercise
44. Increases the number of open capillaries during exercise as opposed to rest
45. Improves blood flow to the active muscles at the peak of training
46. Enhances the functioning of the cardiovascular system
47. Improves efficiency in breathing
48. Lessens sensitivity to the buildup of CO_2
49. Improves breathing—less ventilation is required per liter of O_2 consumption
50. Decreases the chances of the development of osteoporosis
51. Improves the development and strength of connective tissue
52. Increases strength of ligaments
53. Is inversely related to obesity, diabetes, arthritis, and death from cancer
54. Enhances neuromuscular relaxation, thus reducing anxiety and tension
55. Improves resistance to infectious disease
56. Enables you to relax more quickly and completely
57. Alleviates depression
58. Improves emotional stability
59. Enhances clarity of the mind
60. Makes you feel good
61. Increases efficiency of your sweat glands
62. Makes you better able to stay warm in colder environments
63. Improves your body composition
64. Increases bone density
65. Helps you decrease fat tissue more easily
66. Helps you achieve a more agile body
67. Increases your positive attitude about yourself and life
68. Increases the level of the hormone norepinephrine—boosts the spirits
69. Increases the body's level of endorphins—boosts the spirits
70. Stimulates hormonal releases, which relieve pain
71. Alleviates constipation
72. Increases the efficiency of utilizing adrenaline, resulting in more energy
73. Enables you to meet new friends and develop fulfilling relationships
74. Lets you socialize while getting in shape at the same time
75. Helps you move past self-imposed limitations
76. Gives you a greater appreciation for life as a result of feeling better about yourself
77. Enables you to better enjoy all types of physical activities
78. Makes the clothes you wear look better on you
79. Improves athletic performance

80. Makes you feel more sensual
81. Improves the whole quality of your life
82. May add a few years to your life
83. Increases your range of motion
84. Gives you a feeling of control or mastery over your life
85. Stimulates and improves concentration
86. Decreases appetite when you work out 20–60 minutes
87. Gets your mind off of irritations and annoyances
88. Stimulates a feeling of well-being and accomplishment
89. Revitalizes and invigorates the body and mind
90. Is a wonderful way to enjoy nature and the great outdoors
91. Increases the body's own awareness of itself
92. Reduces or precludes boredom
93. Makes it possible to keep up with your children
94. Increases your ability to solve problems more easily and often effortlessly
95. Gives you a clearer perspective on ideas, issues, problems, and challenges
96. Helps you sleep better at night and feel more rested in the morning
97. Integrates body, mind, and spirit
98. Is a great activity for the family to do together
99. Increases libido and enjoyment of sex
100. Affords you the opportunity to experience your fullest potential
101. Is the best way to enjoy and celebrate life

I could list many more, but I think you get the picture. One of the best overall benefits of exercise is the opportunity it offers you to add discipline to your life, to show the power of setting goals and keeping commitments, and seeing your dreams come to fruition.

Please refer to page 217 for more information on how to order one of my favorite pieces of exercise equipment for your home or office—a rebounder.

❄ ✳ ❄

THE HEALING POWER
OF SILENCE & SOLITUDE

"Seek time to be alone;
and in the cave of inner silence,
you shall find the wellspring of wisdom."

— PARAMAHANSA YOGANANDA

No one disputes that regular exercise and a wholesome diet are essential ingredients for being radiantly healthy and living a balanced, vibrant life. But I believe there are other equally important elements that are often overlooked. In the pursuit of our physical goals such as a strong, fit, well-toned, healthy body, we often neglect the importance of nurturing the emotional and spiritual sides of our being, from which true happiness, peace, and fulfillment emanate. To sustain these aspects of ourselves, two processes are tops on my list—*solitude* and *silence.*

It was Paramahansa Yogananda who said: "We should not allow noise and sensory activities to tear down the ladder of our inner attention, because we are listening for the footsteps of God to come into our body temple." I love that thought. Noise certainly seems to be part of our everyday lives—from the alarm clock in the morning to the traffic outside and the never-ending sounds of voices, radio, and television. Our bodies and minds appear acclimated to these outside intrusions—or are they?

Two decades ago, the Committee on Environmental Quality of the Federal Council for Science and Technology found that "growing numbers of researchers fear the dangerous and hazardous effects of intense noise on human health are seriously underestimated." Similarly, the late Vice President Nelson Rockefeller noted that when people are fully aware of the damage that noise can inflict on man, "peace and quiet will surely rank along with clean skies and pure waters as top priorities for our generation."

In his terrific book *Save Your Hearing Now,* Michael D. Seidman, M.D., FACS, writes that more recent studies suggest that we pay a price for adapting to noise: increased blood pressure, heart rate, and adrenaline secretion; heightened aggression; impaired resistance to disease; and a sense of helplessness. Research indicates that when we can control noise, however, its effects are much less damaging.

Sounds of Silence

While I haven't been able to find any studies on the effects of quiet in repairing the stress of noise, I know intuitively that most of us love tranquility and need it desperately. We are so used to sound in our lives that its absence can sometimes feel awkward and unsettling. On vacation, for instance, when a soft hush prevails, we may have trouble sleeping. But choosing times of silence can enrich the quality of our lives tremendously. If we find ourselves overworked, stressed out, irritated, or tense, rather than heading for a coffee or snack break, maybe all we need is a "silence break."

Everyone at some time has experienced the feeling of being overwhelmed by life. We all, too, have felt the need to escape, to find a quiet, secluded place to experience the peace of spirit and to be alone with our thoughts. Creating times of silence takes commitment and discipline. Most often, they must be scheduled into the day's activities or we'll never have any.

Maybe you can carve out periods of quiet while at home, where you can be without radio, television, telephones, or voices. If you live with family members, the best option may be early in the morning before the others arise. In that calm, you can become more aware of, and more sensitive to, your surroundings and more in touch with the wholeness of life.

Solitude

From quiet time, you'll recognize the importance of being alone. Silence and solitude go hand in hand. In them, you reconnect with yourself. Being solitary helps clear your channels, fosters peace, and brings spiritual lucidity. When you retreat from the outside world to go within, you can dwell at the very center of yourself and reacquaint yourself with your spiritual nature—the essence of your being and all life.

Outside noise tends to drown out the inner life—the music of the soul. Only in silence and solitude can we go within and nurture our spiritual lives. Within each of us, there's a silence waiting to be embraced. It's the harbor of the heart. When you rediscover that haven, your life will never be the same. In the Bible we read, "There is silence in heaven" (Revelation 8:1) and "For God alone my soul waits in silence" (Psalm 62:1).

Mystics, saints, and spiritual leaders have advocated periods of silence and solitude for spiritual growth. Saint John of the Cross wrote that only in silence can the soul hear the divine; Jesus prayed much by himself and spent long hours in wordless communion with God. Gandhi devoted every Monday to a day of silence, in which he was better able to meditate and pray, to seek within himself the solutions to all of the problems and responsibilities that he carried. When I read about his practice several years ago, I was so inspired and moved that I decided to adopt a similar discipline in my life. So now one day each week, for two consecutive days once a month, and for several days in a row at each change of season, I spend time in solitude, silence, prayer, and fasting.

"You long for peace. You think of peace as being goodwill towards each other, goodwill among the nations, the laying down of arms. But peace is far more than this; it can only be understood and realized within your heart. It lies beneath all the turmoil and noise and clamor of the world, beneath feeling, beneath thought. It is found in the deep, deep silence and stillness of the soul. It is spirit: it is God," writes White Eagle in one of my all-time favorite books, *The Quiet Mind.* Invite quiet and solitude into your life, and find that place within you where peace and stillness reside.

How do you feel about being alone? It's quite different from loneliness. In the book *The Courage to Be,* Paul Tillich expressed this idea beautifully when he wrote the following: "Our language has wisely sensed the two sides of being alone. It has created the word *loneliness* to express the pain of being alone. And it has created the word *solitude* to express the glory of being alone."

Loneliness is something you do to yourself. Have you ever experienced it even when you're with other people? We're so used to being around others and so unaccustomed to being by ourselves that we have, in a sense, become "a people" and not persons. We must reclaim ourselves and reconnect with our wholeness and the peace of solitude.

Choose to Make Solitude Your Friend

Everyone needs times of privacy and solitude. In my counseling, I always encourage couples to spend occasional time alone—not only daily, but also at regular intervals during the week, month, and year. In this way, you regain your identity as individuals. You bring so much more to the marriage when you come from feeling whole, complete, and strong, and spending time on your own fosters these qualities.

With a little creativity, a marriage can accommodate solitude and privacy. I've witnessed all types of arrangements, including separate vacations, private rooms in the house, living apart during the week and coming together on weekends, and having special times during the day during which each person is left in peace.

I know several individuals who do everything possible to keep from being alone. Often this is because they've never tried it, they're afraid of loneliness, or they're simply uncomfortable with themselves. They haven't yet discovered the peace of their own company. It's not scary to be by yourself—it's absolutely wonderful! Loneliness isn't a state of being; it's a state of mind, which you can choose to change.

I realize that I live differently from most in that I go to great lengths to secure my time of solitude and privacy. It's a great comfort to me to be by myself; it's like returning home to an old friend or lover after being away too long. This isn't a luxury; it is a right and a necessity.

Through the years, I've gone on several vision quests. These are periods of solitude during which you can take time for looking into your soul, finding a new direction or path, or simply reconnecting with your Higher Self. On these occasions, I usually go to the mountains or the ocean for prayer, meditation, fasting, reflection, and being alone. I spend much of my time outdoors, open to the beauty and love all around me. On this peaceful, reflective retreat, the earth, sky, wind, animals, incredible beauty, and divine order of everything take on a new and personal meaning. I commune with the trees, moon, flowers, and animals. My vision quests always show me that the most profound lessons in life come through nature, solitude, and silence.

It's my contention that all of the other good things we endeavor to provide for ourselves—including sound nutrition, daily exercise, and material wealth—will be of reduced value unless we learn to live in harmony with ourselves, which means knowing ourselves and finding peace in our own company. This serenity is a natural occurrence of spending quiet time without others. When we do so, we realize that we're never really alone and that we can live more fully by focusing on inner guidance rather than on external things.

Embrace solitude. Walk in silence among the trees, in the mountains, by the ocean, and with the sun and moon as your friends. Be by yourself and experience a whole new way of celebrating yourself and life. Feel the heartbeat of silence; bathe in its light and love. Know within yourself that you're a child of God, and in your silence is Heaven.

When from our better selves we have too long
Been parted by the hurrying world, and droop,
Sick of its business, of its pleasures tired,
How gracious, how benign, is Solitude . . .

— WILLIAM WORDSWORTH

❋ ❋ ❋

THE HEALING POWER
OF LOVE

This story, which I call "The Butterfly and the Skater," illustrates how the power of love can transcend time and place.

While my mom may no longer be in my life physically, she's doubtless with me through my loving memories and will always hold the most cherished place in my heart. We share a loving connection that transcends appearances. I thought you might enjoy reading about an experience I had that showed me that Mom is closer to me now than ever before.

Alone and pensive, I was in-line skating along the beach, oblivious to the laughter of late beachgoers, the people passing me on the bike path, and even the sunset over Santa Monica Bay that illuminated the sky and water with luscious colors. A palpable sadness infused every cell in my body. I was grieving the loss of my best friend and inspiration—my mom; she had died of cancer just one week before. We shared a love for butterflies, and shortly before she passed away, she told me that whenever I saw a butterfly in the future, it would be Mom, reminding me that she'll always be in my heart. During my workout that day, I was missing her so much that I could hardly breathe, and the continual flow of tears made it difficult to navigate on the path.

And then it happened. What felt like a gigantic rock—it actually was only a quarter-sized stone—caught a wheel of my skate, and down I went, slamming into the concrete. Fortunately, no one was around to see my less-than-graceful descent, except for a woman sitting on a bench nearby. She immediately came over to make sure I was okay. Her gentle kindness and amiable countenance immediately comforted me. Seeing the jagged lacerations on my helmet, resulting from my skid on the pathway, I was feeling grateful that I'd worn protective gear. I really was fine, except for minor scratches and abrasions on my arms and legs and some major bruises to my pride.

As I got myself under control and realized that I could skate back to my car, I focused on the sympathetic woman by my side and noticed her clothing for the first time. She was wearing a brilliant butterfly shirt and a large-brimmed hat teeming with colorful straw butterflies. Until that moment, I'd forgotten what my mom had told me about "butterfly sightings," and I experienced full-body angel bumps (aka goose bumps). When I asked my Good Samaritan her name, she replied as she removed her hat, "My name is June, but my close friends call me 'Wings,' because of my love for these magnificent winged insects." The angel bumps on my body intensified: My mom's name was June.

I felt moved to tell "Wings" about my wonderful mother and that talk we had shortly before she slipped into a coma. Before I could finish the story, an exquisite periwinkle butterfly fluttered in front of us and landed on the back of my hand. Speechless, we both drank in this wonderful experience. I knew my mom was letting me know that she was well and happy and would always be with me in her special way. I lifted up my hand, brought the motionless butterfly close to my face, and celebrated its presence in my life. Moments later, it floated away, and for the first time in a week, I cried tears of joy, not sadness.

❋ ❋ ❋

The Healing Power
of Salubrious Green Smoothies

"In general, mankind . . .
eat about twice as much as nature requires."

— Benjamin Franklin

Is your day filled with endless activities and "busyness" from morning to night? Do you wish you had more time to spend in your kitchen preparing healthful meals? Have you ever longed for a delicious and nutritious meal that would take only minutes to make and seconds to clean up? Or have you wondered what you could have for a snack that would satisfy you, yet not overburden your body and digestive tract with too many calories? Well, you're in luck today because I have a perfect solution to all of these quandaries. Enter *Salubrious Smoothies*.

I love the adjective *salubrious,* which means "favorable to or promoting health or well-being." An apt synonym is *healthful.* So this melodious word—*salubrious*—beautifully describes my special green smoothies. Before highlighting their benefits, let's first explore the importance of eating sufficient amounts of fresh produce.

In a recent review of 206 human epidemiological studies, compared with all other beneficial foods, green vegetables showed the strongest protective effect against cancer, heart disease, arthritis, diabetes, obesity, and high blood pressure. Unfortunately, only one American in 500 gets enough calories from vegetables to ensure this defense.

Indubitably, high green-vegetable consumption is associated with powerful protection against disease. That is why the cornerstone of a heart-healthy, cancer-protective, and longevity-favorable diet is to eat as many raw and steamed green vegetables as you can. The more of these nutrient-rich foods you consume, the higher your diet will be in nutrient density. What's more, many vegetables contain *more protein* per calorie than meat, and many have more calcium per calorie than milk. For example, romaine lettuce is a rich powerhouse containing hundreds of cancer-fighting phytonutrients; it gets 50 percent of its calories from protein and 18 percent from unsaturated fat. Kale is even higher in protein and has more than 20 percent more calcium per calorie than milk.

If you eat like most Americans, or even if you follow the USDA's food pyramid recommendations precisely (6–11 servings of bread, rice, and pasta made from grains and 4–6 servings of dairy, meat, poultry, or fish), you're eating a diet high in calories, with dangerous levels of saturated fat. To create vibrant health, you need to eschew or reduce all processed junk foods and products made with white flour, white sugar, artificial colorings, additives, and other chemicals. Moreover, you must consume at least 7–12 servings of fresh fruits and vegetables daily.

Blended Salads

For some, eating so much produce is hard to stomach (I couldn't resist the pun) or to fit into a busy lifestyle. Here's my solution: Blend your salad. Before you turn up your nose at this suggestion or perhaps turn the page before finishing this section, I want to encourage you to give it a try. Blended salads really do make a particularly healthful, delectable dish and are quick and easy to make. I eat them frequently. For example, I often take baby romaine lettuce and blend it with a banana, an apple, and a couple of dates. These salubrious smoothies (to use the term I coined) enable me to consume four to six ounces of raw leafy greens quickly and easily and to glean their powerful health effects. They taste great, too, and what I definitely appreciate is that cleanup takes seconds!

Blending salad vegetables, especially leafy greens, with some fresh fruit and water, tea, or fresh juice makes a resplendently green, luscious smoothie. Raw greens are "wonder foods" for your health, and when you consume them in this form, you get more of their powerful nutrients. The blades of the blender break down the cell walls, dramatically increasing the bioavailability of the nutrients. This means that these beverages are easy to digest. Simply put, when blended well, all of the valuable nutrients in these fruits and vegetables are divided into such small particles that it becomes easy for the body to assimilate the nutrients. They start to get absorbed in your mouth.

Green smoothies, as opposed to juices, are a complete food because they still have fiber—and they're an excellent healthful meal or snack for both adults and children. When whipping up these salutary blends (a daily activity for me), I always make extra and offer it to my friends or clients. Some of them still eat a standard American diet. Yet when they finish their big glass or bowl of my salubrious smoothie, they're always pleasantly surprised by how wonderful it is. To date, I've never had anyone tell me that they didn't like how it tasted.

By drinking two to three cups of green smoothies daily, you'll consume almost enough greens to nourish your body, and they'll be well assimilated. You'll be getting raw, enzyme- and nutrient-rich blends of fresh fruits and vegetables. Moreover, they help heal, detoxify, and rejuvenate your body; accelerate fat loss; and restore youthful vitality. I'm often told by newcomers to these beverages that after a couple of weeks of drinking them, they've lost their appetite for junk and processed foods and have actually begun to hunger for more greens.

To make these salad smoothies, you must start with a top-quality blender and juicer.

The Best Blender

Known as the gold standard of all blenders and made by the industry king, Blendtec, the one I use and recommend is called *The Total Blender*. Recently, it was highlighted in a special presentation on HGTV as one of the hottest new products and innovations in housewares design at the International Home & Housewares Show in Chicago. It's indispensable in my kitchen, cuisine classes around the country, and private culinary instruction. Several times each day, this easy-to-use blender helps me create a variety of mouthwatering dishes. For more information on The Total Blender and why it's the grand prix of all blenders, please visit: **www.SusanSmithJones.com** and click on *Susan's Favorite Products*.

The Best Juicer

There are many fruit and vegetable juicers on the market, but for the highest quality, I always recommend the Champion 2000+ Juicer. It makes preparing fresh, wholesome fruit and vegetable juices a joy.

One of the best known and most popular worldwide, the Champion 2000+ Juicer includes a number of features that bring the power and durability of commercial juicers directly to your kitchen countertop. Delicious fruit and vegetable beverages of the highest quality have never been easier to prepare. Juice from the Champion is darker, richer in color, and contains more of the nutrients you desire than that produced by other machines.

Two reasons why I use the Champion are:

1. It is easy to clean.
2. It does much more than make juice.

In fact, it's the ultimate multitasking culinary machine. I use it to make fruit sauces and purées; sorbets, sherbets, and "ice cream" (from frozen fruit); baby foods; and creamy nut butters. The Champion 2000+ also functions as a grain mill, allowing me to quickly and easily prepare healthful, hearty whole grains.

For more information, please visit: **www.SusanSmithJones.com** and click on *Susan's Favorite Products*. To order, visit: **www.championjuicer.com** or call: (866) WE JUICE (935-8423).

Making Salubrious Smoothies

Green smoothies consist of a combination of greens, fruit, and water or another liquid base. With a ratio of approximately 60/40 of fruits to veggies, the fruit taste dominates the flavor, yet the green vegetables balance out that sweetness, adding a delectable zest.

While I often use water as a base, I also use a variety of other liquids that you may want to consider, too. For example, I always have pitchers filled with chilled fresh tea in my refrigerator. They might be individual flavors such as peppermint or chamomile, or they might be combinations with flavors that I enjoy. These make a delicious, no-calorie addition.

To make my smoothies richer and higher in protein, I might use *Living Harvest Hemp Milk* (vanilla, chocolate, or original) or any of the nut milks that I always have freshly made in the refrigerator. These take only minutes to prepare and add creaminess to the smoothie. (For more recipes, please refer to my books *The Healing Power of NatureFoods* and *Be Healthy~Stay Balanced*.)

I make fresh juice in my Champion juicer to use in smoothies, but if you don't have time, I also use and recommend a variety of different antioxidant-rich beverages available in the natural-food stores and even in better supermarkets. For example, I always have kombucha drinks on hand, as well as 100 percent fresh juices made from blueberry, raspberry, açai, goji, passion fruit, cranberry, guava, mango, and others chilled in my refrigerator. Just ½ cup added to the smoothie increases the nutritional benefit and ever so slightly changes the color and taste.

Some of my favorite greens to use when making salubrious smoothies include parsley, spinach, romaine, celery, cucumber, and kale. Because they're delicious and plentiful in protein and many other nutrients, I also use sunflower-seed green sprouts.

My favorite fruits for these beverages include pears, peaches, nectarines, bananas, mangoes, kiwi, strawberries, raspberries, fresh figs, and apples. Ripe bananas and pitted dates also make the perfect sweeteners. Blueberries work well, flavor- and nutrient-wise, and their color transforms the smoothie from green to a darker blue-purple.

Favorite Food Combinations

The following are some combinations I make most often. Simply blend until smooth and enjoy. Each provides one to two servings, depending on whether I'd like a meal or a snack. When I want the smoothie to be sweeter, I use one or more pitted medjool dates, raw agave nectar, a chunk or more of banana (fresh or frozen), date sugar, or maple syrup. If you want the smoothie to be thicker and richer in omega-3 fatty acids, just add a tablespoon or two of flaxseed meal and/or reduce the liquid.

If I want to increase the protein, I add *Organic Hemp Protein* powders and seeds by Living Harvest or cashew, almond, walnut, or sunflower-seed milk. Most of the time, however, I just use raw fresh fruits and vegetables and add some water, tea, or freshly made juice as the base.

All of the smoothies can also be poured in a bowl instead of a glass, and eaten as a chilled or room-temperature soup. In a white dish, the colorful blends are dazzling. Be inventive and have fun in your creations.

A Few Sample Recipes

I intentionally didn't make the following recipes too exact. I encourage you to experiment with amounts and try different combinations according to what fresh (preferably organic) produce you have on hand. In place of water, I often substitute some kind of tea that's already made and chilled in my refrigerator. Additionally, when it's warm or hot outside, I enjoy using frozen fruit or adding three to four ice cubes.

The sky's the limit with what you can create when making these nutrient-dense, green, salubrious smoothies. Experiment on your own, and within no time, you'll be an expert. Here are three of my favorite blends to pique your interest. In the Recipes section of this book, you'll find lots more of these mouth-watering taste sensations.

Strawberry-Banana-Romaine Smoothie

1 cup strawberries
2 bananas
4–6 romaine lettuce leaves
½ cup water or juice

Place ingredients in a blender with some of the liquid. Blend, adding additional liquid if necessary.

Apple-Kale-Lemon Smoothie

4 apples
4–5 kale leaves
Juice of ½ lemon
½ cup water or juice

Place ingredients in a blender with some of the liquid. Blend, adding additional liquid if necessary.

Kiwi-Banana-Celery Smoothie

4 kiwis
1 banana
3 stalks celery
¾ cup water or juice

Place ingredients in a blender with some of the liquid. Blend, adding additional liquid if necessary.

PART IV

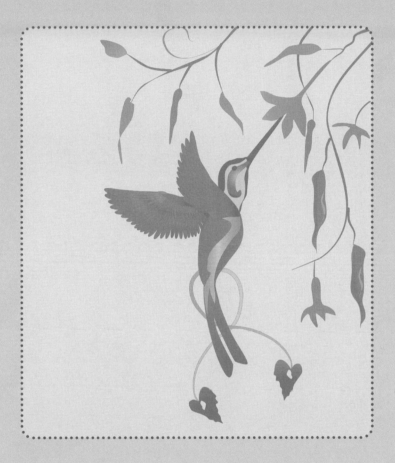

MORE ENTRÉES

50 NatureFoods: Part II

"The more you eat, the less flavor.
The less you eat, the more flavor."

— Chinese proverb

Let's continue with our perusal of the 50 revitalizing NatureFoods that will help you along on the path to better health, wellness, and vitality, qualities that can greatly enhance your self-esteem and enjoyment of life.

Please keep in mind that while I'm certainly singing the praises of these best-of-the-best foods and describing their extraordinary characteristics, *all* fresh fruits, vegetables, legumes, raw nuts and seeds, and whole grains bring tremendous benefits. The unsurpassed nutrients and other qualities I describe for individual foods also are found to varying degrees in *all* of the NatureFoods I recommend for a complete, overall healthful diet.

Go Green

As you can see, we have a "green" theme going on in this book. It's the color of nature, and in my estimation, the color of health. When you're green inside, you're healthy and clean inside. So "think green."

The United States is an industrialized nation, where far fewer people go to bed hungry than in the many developing areas around the globe. But would you believe that as a whole, we're a very malnourished country? While we may be eating three square meals each day, most people aren't providing their bodies with the nutrients they need to boost their natural defense system and keep them healthy. According to the Organization for Economic Cooperation and Development (OECD), the United States has the highest percentage of health-care costs spent on pharmaceuticals in the world ("OECD Health Data 2005: How Does the United States Compare?" Organization for Economic Cooperation and Development). With that said, *isn't it time we start thinking about how to maintain our good health instead of waiting until something compromises it?*

Since what we put into our bodies plays a major role in how we act and feel, let's examine what types of foods will help promote and maintain good health all year round.

The term *go green* has grown massively popular as of late, due to increased awareness of environmental issues and the need for immediate changes in the way we treat our precious planet. Well, much like our Earth needs "green" (that is, trees and plants), our bodies require it as well—from green foods! If you're wondering what the common denominator is between the things that help heal and maintain the ecology of the planet and those that do the same for our bodies, the answer is *chlorophyll*. While I have an entire category devoted to the substance, it's so important that I'm going to talk about it some more here—approaching it from another angle, if you will—in the hopes that you'll start today and consume as much green food as possible.

At the root of green life on Earth is the process of photosynthesis. Through photosynthesis, these plants use chlorophyll to adjust the energy of the sun and the nutrients in their environment into their own growth, and then bring that power to countless other creatures in the form of plant foods. Thus, the difference between life and death on Earth is the presence of green plants. Chlorophyll literally transforms light into life! The benefits of this substance on the human body include renewing damaged tissue, building blood, fighting off harmful germs and microorganisms, helping facilitate wound healing, increasing healthful intestinal flora, improving liver function and gum health, and triggering enzymes that produce vitamins E, A, and K.

As previously mentioned, in a review of 206 human epidemiological studies, the foods that revealed the strongest protective benefit against cancer, heart disease, arthritis, diabetes, obesity, and high blood pressure were green vegetables. Unfortunately, just one in 500 Americans consumes enough calories from vegetables to ensure this defense. The cornerstone of your new heart-healthy, cancer-protective, longevity-favorable diet is to eat as many raw and steamed green vegetables as you can. The more of these foods you eat, the higher your diet will be in nutrient density.

My grandmother Fritzie was right when she told me to eat my greens. These foods are detoxifying, rejuvenating, and renewing. If you want to heal your body, accelerate fat loss, and look younger, get more greens!

Fast-growing plants, such as wheat, barley, and alfalfa cereal grasses, contain rich sources of chlorophyll. You'll read more about these in the pages of this book. Chlorella is another superb NatureFood with oodles of chlorophyll. You'll also find quality chlorophyll and a treasure trove of nutrients in spinach, parsley, and sea vegetables, to name a few.

Eating two large salads and extra servings of vegetables each day helps you get enough greens to bolster your health. But not everyone has the time to eat several servings, so here's another NatureFood that's teeming with green goodness and a myriad of nutrients that you might want to consider adding to your diet, as I have for years—*Aphanizomenon flos-aquae (AFA)*.

For thousands of years, algae have been used worldwide as an excellent food source and potent medicine. For 25 years, the naturally occurring AFA growing in Oregon has been harvested and sold as a unique dietary supplement that's teeming with health-promoting compounds. "Although AFA grows in many other areas of the world," writes Christian Drapeau, M.Sc., in his book, *Primordial Food Aphanizomenon flos-aquae: A Wild Blue-Green Alga with Unique Health Properties,* "the biomass that accumulates every year in Klamath Lake is unique in its abundance as well as its purity."

E3Live is 100 percent AFA. It's available in its complete fresh-frozen liquid form. It's collected only from the deepest, most primitive waters of Klamath Lake and harvested only at peak times of optimal growth, when the AFA is the heartiest, healthiest, and most vibrant. For more than 12 years, I've taken E3Live consistently, and I highly recommend it to everyone. It provides more chlorophyll than wheatgrass; 60 percent high-quality protein; all of the B vitamins, including B_{12}; essential omega-3 and omega-6 fatty acids; and powerful digestive enzymes. It's also organic, kosher, vegan, raw, and versatile.

World-renowned holistic physician/psychiatrist and author of several books, including *Conscious Eating,* Dr. Gabriel Cousens says this about E3Live: "As a physician working with thousands of clients, I find that E3Live helps to restore overall biochemical balance by nourishing the body at the cellular level. The positive response from the use of E3Live has been extraordinary. E3Live has the potential to enhance every aspect of our lives—mind, body, and soul."

I encourage you to try it for 90 days . . . just one season, and see for yourself how great you'll feel and look. For more information, please visit: **www.SusanSmithJones. com** and click on *Susan's Favorite Products*. To order, visit: **www.E3Live.com** or call: (888) 800-7070 or (541) 273-2212.

Grapes & Raisins

Grapes were first cultivated about 7,000 years ago by the Egyptians. New varieties were developed by the Greeks and Romans and eventually introduced into Europe. Grapes are now a crop on six of the seven continents. Most of the 60 million tons grown annually worldwide are fermented to produce wine, but you don't need to drink it to derive protection. Red grapes offer similar benefits. The fruit is also made into jams and spreads, used in cooking, and eaten raw as a snack food.

Low in calories, grapes are favored for their sweet, juicy flavor. Another reason to eat these valuable beauties may be found in research on the disease prevention role of bioflavonoids and other plant chemicals. Anthocyanins found in red and purple grapes have numerous health benefits, including lowering heart disease and cancer risk.

The fruits contain quercetin, a plant pigment that is thought to regulate the levels of blood cholesterol and also reduce the action of platelets, blood cells that are instrumental in forming clots. Some researchers theorize that it's the quercetin that lowers the risk of heart attack among moderate wine drinkers.

Grapes contain ellagic acid, which is thought to protect the lungs against environmental toxins. They also naturally have salicylates, compounds similar to the major ingredient in aspirin. Salicylates have an anticlotting effect and may also account for the benefits of wine with respect to heart disease. (People who are allergic to aspirin may react to grapes and grape products, too.) The skin of grapes contains resveratrol, a phytochemical linked to a reduction of heart disease, as well as a lowered risk of cancer or stroke.

Dieters and those with a slow metabolism will especially enjoy freshly squeezed grape juice because it stimulates metabolic rate. Its flavonoids are among the most powerful antioxidants around—maybe even better than vitamins C or E. In your body, flavonoids help prevent LDL cholesterol from oxidizing (the process that enables cholesterol to stick to your artery walls and create blockages). Grape juice is also a source of potassium, with eight ounces providing about 335 mg. When grapes are in season, I buy pounds of organically grown red or purple varieties, juice them, and freeze the liquid into cubes that I drop into my water, teas, or fresh fruit juices. (Store the cubes in plastic freezer bags.) I also freeze washed seedless grapes whole; they make a wonderful treat on hot summer days.

To reap the full benefit of grapes, it's best to select red or purple varieties because they seem to contain the highest concentration of healthful compounds. Also go organic, if possible. Commercially grown fruits are usually sprayed with pesticides and treated with sulfur dioxide to preserve their color and extend shelf life. This NatureFood should always be washed well before being eaten.

Raisins, dried grapes, can help improve digestion and keep blood healthy. If you have high blood pressure (or even if you don't, but you want to make sure your pressure stays in a healthy range), raisins are one of the best snacks you can buy because of their high level of potassium—1,090 mg in a cup. Raisins are a highly concentrated source of other nutrients and calories—one cup contains a whopping 440 calories while providing three grams of iron and six grams of fiber.

It takes about 4½ pounds of fresh grapes to produce one pound of raisins. Black raisins are actually dried in the sun, which gives them their dark, shriveled look. They're used for both baking and snacking. Golden seedless raisins are exposed to the fumes of burning sulfur in a closed chamber, which gives them their golden hue. They're usually used in baking—in fruitcakes, for example—because of their attractive appearance. I encourage you to buy organic raisins because of the high levels of pesticides used in growing grapes.

Better yet, do what I do; dry them yourself in a low-temperature food dehydrator. (I use the best food dehydrator on the market, the *Excalibur,* **www. drying123.com**; see the Resources section for more information.) Raisins that you dry yourself are a special delight for your taste buds. They also make much-appreciated gifts.

Green Beans

Also known as snap beans, these are among the most common vegetables grown and eaten in North America. The legumes are grown for their pods, which are picked while young, when the seeds are still small and tender. There are more than 150 varieties in cultivation today, including thick runner beans, the more slender French beans, and the yellow wax beans.

Compared to most other vegetables, green beans age quickly once harvested, so plan to use them right away. They're delicious eaten raw; or they can be blanched or steamed; served on their own; or used in salads, casseroles, soups, and stir-fries—either whole, cut into lengths, or sliced into small rounds. For French style (cut into ribbon-thin lengths), trim the beans and use a vegetable peeler with a frenching end to cut them into thin strands. This works best with very fresh beans.

Select vegetables that are firm, whole, and crisp, without rust spots. A fresh bean snaps crisply and feels velvety to the touch, while old ones are bulging and leathery. Those with greatest commercial availability include plain green beans, Italian (flat Romano), purple podded, wax beans (which are usually yellow), and yard-long beans.

Fresh green beans are rich in vitamins A and B complex, calcium, and potassium. You'll also find that they're good sources of folate, magnesium, and vitamin C. They've long been considered a diuretic and beneficial in treating diabetes. With their abundance of potassium, they supply the alkaline needs of the pancreas and salivary glands. Note that the yellow (wax) bean is considered inferior to the green bean in nutritional value.

Next time you're making fresh vegetable juice at home in your juicer, throw in a few of these green beauties. You'll reap the benefits of their nutrients, and you'll get extra chlorophyll to boot. I also cut green beans into thin strips (or in half) and dry them at a low temperature in my Excalibur food dehydrator. They make a tasty treat, especially when seasoned with some herbs and spices.

Herbs & Spices

On these pages, I've grouped together eight great foods under the general heading of Herbs & Spices. What we often think of as simple, recipe-enhancing plants also have led long, distinguished lives as healers. Basil, delicious when paired with fresh tomatoes, has served for centuries to settle stomachs. Parsley, a color enhancer for mashed potatoes and an enlivener of hummus, has long been used to banish bloating and freshen breath. Thyme, a familiar fragrance on roasted vegetables, has revealed its anti-ulcer powers in the lab. Ginger, used frequently in teas, is a consummate herb to reduce all kinds of inflammation, digestive distress, and nausea such as morning and motion sickness.

Cinnamon may be the best-known, best-loved spice in America, but until recently few people knew that it also was a serious medicine because of its ability to improve insulin function, lower blood sugar, and help keep blood healthy. I like cinnamon in my morning orange juice, but it's also excellent on most fruits and oatmeal. The yellow spice turmeric, a constituent of curry powder, contains high concentrations of the potent antioxidant curcumin, which, according to new studies, helps stifle cancer.

If you see your spices only as a way to make your food more flavorful, it's time to take a closer look. (See page 217 for *free* samples.)

— **Basil:** This beautiful green herb often turns up in Shakespeare's plays as a remedy for colds and headaches. More recently, studies have shown that fresh leaves aid digestion and lower blood-sugar levels. Add torn leaves to salads and tomato dishes, or chop and grind them into pesto in a food processor. One of the many reasons I enjoy using it in as many dishes as possible is because in Italy, basil is a sign of love!

— **Cinnamon:** Most people love the taste of this one. Its fragrance conjures up thoughts of the holidays and special treats for the taste buds. An ancient spice obtained from the dried bark of two Asian evergreens, cinnamon is a highly versatile flavoring, as well as a carminative that relieves bloating and gas.

Adding cinnamon to foods, especially sugary ones, helps normalize blood sugar by making insulin more sensitive. The spice's most active ingredient is methyl hydroxy chalcone polymer (MHCP), which increases the processing of blood sugar by 2,000 percent. So using cinnamon in tiny amounts—even sprinkled in desserts—makes insulin more efficient. Cloves, turmeric, and bay leaves also work, but they're weaker. Avoiding high circulating levels of blood sugar and insulin may help ward off diabetes and obesity. Steady lower insulin levels are also an indication of slower aging and greater longevity.

Here's an easy way to get on the cinnamon bandwagon and reap all of the benefits. You've probably heard about putting slices of lemon, lime, or cucumbers in your water to rev up the taste; next time, add a cinnamon stick. That's right! It adds a delicious, subtle flavor that's quite wonderful, and you can use the same stick for about two days before replacing it with a new one.

Most mornings, I fill my 64-ounce glass pitcher with fresh, purified water and add one to two cinnamon sticks. From this one vessel, I transfer my water into glasses or bottles to take with me, so I'm always keeping myself well hydrated and energetically sound. My grandmother Fritzie taught me to do this, and it's a delightful way to enjoy this fragrant and nutritionally rich culinary spice. Next time you're carrying a bottle filled with H_2O, put a cinnamon stick in it. If nothing else, it's a great conversation piece.

Most days, I also find ways to include cinnamon in my meals. I sprinkle it on fruits and cereal; blend it in smoothies; and incorporate it in fruit sauces, purées, soups, and squash dishes. Don't forget to put cinnamon sticks in your tea or other hot beverages, too.

Here's one of my favorite breakfast or snack treats. I start with a generous amount of cut-up, crisp romaine lettuce on a plate. Then on top of the lettuce, I combine large diced sections of pink or red grapefruit, orange, and kiwi; I sprinkle cinnamon over them. Absolutely delicious, and because of the high water content of the food, it's very detoxifying and rejuvenating. (You can substitute any of your favorite fruits.) I also make sachets of cinnamon, nutmeg, and cloves for gifts to hang in the kitchen, closets, the linen cupboard, or the laundry room.

— **Fennel seeds:** The ancient Greeks ate this aromatic herb to suppress their hunger. All parts of the plant are used in cooking, but the most potent medicinal properties are in the seeds. An infusion of them (one teaspoon of crushed seeds added to one cup of boiled water, steeped for five minutes, then strained) eases flatulence and colic in young children and prevents heartburn and indigestion in adults.

— **French tarragon:** Native to southern Europe, this great culinary herb is milder than its pungent Russian cousin (which is simply called "tarragon"). French tarragon has a light anise-seed flavor and combines perfectly with rice and vegetables. A tea made from the herb will aid digestion and help relieve insomnia and constipation. To make the tea, steep one teaspoon of dried leaves in one cup of freshly boiled water, covered, for five to ten minutes. Strain.

— **Oregano:** "No wonder oregano has been used since antiquity to fight infection," says Harry G. Preuss, M.D., physiologist at Georgetown University Medical Center and a top researcher in the field of the healing powers of herbs and spices. He found oregano oil as effective as the common antibiotic vancomycin in treating staph infections in mice. It also wiped out an infectious fungus. A daily dose of oregano oil, mixed with oils from fenugreek, cumin, and pumpkin seeds, reduced blood pressure and improved blood sugar and insulin sensitivity in diabetic rats. In Texas research, oregano killed parasites in humans. The point, according to Preuss, is that people who eat small regular doses of oregano may get antibiotic and antidiabetic benefits, although more tests on humans are needed to verify this.

— **Rosemary:** This wonderful culinary herb contains oil of camphor, which gives it a fragrant scent and a pleasantly pungent flavor, sometimes described as a cross between sage and lavender with a touch of ginger. The small, needle-shaped leaves are used fresh; they should be crushed or minced to bring out their full flavor before sprinkling over or rubbing into foods. Whole sprigs can be placed in olive oil for an alternative to butter, and the pale blue flowers make a wonderful addition to salads. Rosemary especially complements the herbs bay, chervil, chives, parsley, and thyme.

Rosemary is high in easily assimilable calcium and benefits the entire nervous system. It helps alleviate depression and eases headaches. Studies also show that this fragrant herb helps with respiratory troubles, corrects and improves the function of the liver and gallbladder, strengthens and tones the muscles of the stomach, acts to raise blood pressure and improve circulation, and even helps with potency disturbances. Its diuretic action is effective in alleviating rheumatism and gout, as well as kidney stones. Rosemary has a long-standing reputation as an invigorating herb, imparting a zest for life that's to some degree reflected in its distinctive taste.

The scent alone is said to preserve youth. (How intoxicating!) World-famous biological researcher Dr. James Duke makes a drink that he says is his own herbal secret for staying mentally sharp. He calls it his "Anti-Alzheimer's Cocktail," made by steeping several sprigs of rosemary in lemonade. Dr. Duke says the antioxidant chemicals in rosemary have a similar effect to those in the latest drugs being used to treat Alzheimer's.

— **Sage:** This remarkable Mediterranean herb is antiseptic, antispasmodic, and antibiotic. It has been used for centuries to treat sore throats, poor digestion, and hormonal problems, and to stimulate the brain. Before cooking with sage leaves, quickly immerse them in hot water; this will bring the leaf oils to the surface and enhance the flavor.

— **Turmeric:** As mentioned previously, turmeric contains curcumin, a potent antioxidant believed to help prevent cancer. In test tubes, 80 percent of malignant prostate cells self-destructed when exposed to curcumin. Feeding mice curcumin dramatically slowed the growth of implanted human-prostate-cancer cells. It may do the same in breast- and colon-cancer cells, researchers say, speculating that it blocks the activation of genes that trigger cancer. Here's another bonus: Curcumin's anti-inflammatory activity reduces arthritic swelling and progressive brain damage in animals. In UCLA research, eating food laced with low doses of the antioxidant slashed Alzheimer's-like plaque in the brains of mice by 50 percent.

Jicama

Pronounced *HEE-kuh-muh* and also known as yam bean and sa kot, this delicious vegetable is native to Mexico and the headwater region of the Amazon in South America. The jicama is the fleshy underground tuber of a member of the legume family. Above ground, this plant is a high-climbing vine with colorful flowers and inedible pea pods. When you find the root in the produce section of your supermarket or natural-food store, it looks like a light brown, oversized turnip with a rough exterior that belies the exquisite, versatile interior. The skin can be peeled easily, revealing a slightly sweet flesh that's similar to water chestnuts—only crunchier.

When shopping for jicama, look for ones that are firm, heavy, and unblemished. If you're going to use them for juicing, be aware that the smaller roots (up to three pounds) are juicier than the larger ones. Store at room temperature for a few days or, if not using right away, refrigerate for up to two weeks. They don't fare well frozen.

A dieter's best friend, the jicama is low in fat, calories, and sodium and is a great source of fiber; calcium; iron; potassium; and vitamins A, B complex, and C. When you're in the mood for something crunchy and slightly sweet, but would prefer to eat a vegetable rather than a fruit, jicama strips just might hit the spot. To me, it tastes like a cross between an apple and a pear. I often take strips of cut-up jicama with me in zip-top bags when I fly so that I have something delicious to munch on. Plain or with a favorite dip, it's always enjoyably satisfying to me.

Don't peel the jicama until just before using it since this vegetable tends to dry out and become hard and fibrous once cut. Because the taste is relatively bland, it lends itself well to almost every type of dish, from fruit medleys and green salads to stir-fries and as a thickener in smoothies. You also can eat it as you would water chestnuts, Jerusalem artichokes, or potatoes; and although its flavor diminishes with cooking, it doesn't lose its crunch. Raw jicama sliced and seasoned with lime juice, salt, and chili pepper is a popular Latin American dish. The root even can be baked like a potato or grated and used as a pie filling.

Lavender

"When my eyes were closed, at night in my little room, my favorite hill used to come to me, and I would sleep under an olive tree, enveloped in the scent of hidden lavender," writes Marcel Pagnol, playwright, novelist, and poet. Those words resonate with me. Every night before I go to sleep, I put a few drops of the essential oil of lavender on my pillow to enjoy its sensuous fragrance and its calming, relaxing effect.

The word *lavender* comes from the Latin *lavare,* "to be washed," because the plant was used in ancient times to perfume bathwater. It originated in the mountainous regions of the Mediterranean and covered vast tracts of dry, barren land in Spain and Italy. A perennial plant with narrow, gray-green leaves and long, purple-flowered spikes, lavender is used to scent sachets, perfumes, and soaps. The dried flowers or sprigs will keep moths away from stored linens and clothes, and the fresh flowers can be rubbed over the skin to deter obnoxious insects.

After a busy, stress-filled day, I'll often make a combination of chamomile and lavender tea because of its calming effect, sipping slowly while I think about the lavender plants beautifying my garden. (In 16th-century England, women and men had the spicy-smelling flowers of lavender quilted into their hats to "comfort the braines.") Taken internally as a tea or culinary herb, lavender is used for indigestion, depression, anxiety, exhaustion, irritability, headaches (including migraines), and bronchial complaints. Its strong scent, like that of mint, is a remedy for dizziness and fainting.

Externally, I use lavender for burns, sunburn, muscular pains, cold sores, and insect bites. Its essential oils contain a substance called *perillyl alcohol* that in laboratory studies has antileukemia and antitumor effects for the liver, pancreas, and breast.

You've probably heard of or used the spice blend characteristic of southern France, *Herbes de Provence.* The distinctive floral essence of lavender is evident in this blend and can easily overpower, so use it sparingly in your meal preparations.

Along with the essential oils of citrus, peppermint, rosemary, and rose, I also keep a bottle of lavender oil in my bathroom and sprinkle a few drops in my bathwater or on the floor of the shower before bathing, depending on my mood and needs.

French chemist René-Maurice Gattefossé discovered lavender's healing powers by accident. While working in his perfume lab in the 1920s, he burned his hand and, in a panic, plunged it into the closest vat, which happened to be filled with lavender oil. When he pulled out his hand, to his surprise and delight, the pain quickly disappeared, and the burn subsequently healed without a trace of a scar.

Lentils

These tiny, disk-shaped legumes grow just one or two to a pod and come in many colors. Numerous varieties are used in Europe, the Middle East, India, and Africa; in the United States, red, brown, and green lentils are the most common. They cook quickly, need no presoaking, and have a distinctive, somewhat peppery flavor. Use them in soups, cook them with other vegetables, or serve them cold in salads. Brown and green lentils hold their shape well after cooking and are excellent for salads; red lentils cook more quickly and work best in purées and other dishes where softness is an advantage. Those sold as *dhal* have had the outer skins removed, and so they're much lower in dietary fiber than other lentils.

Unlike beans, lentils have no sulfur and so produce very little flatulence. They rank just under soy as the top legume protein source. They're high in calcium, magnesium, sodium, potassium, phosphorus, chlorine, and vitamin A. You may want to eat them as a way to help reduce blood cholesterol, control insulin and blood sugar, and lower blood pressure. They contain compounds that inhibit cancer. In addition, they help regulate colon function and may assist in the prevention of hemorrhoids.

Like many Americans, I grew up knowing only one lentil variety—a brown and rather bland-tasting legume. Today, we have a greater selection. India has more than 50 multicolored varieties to choose from, either whole or split and husked. A tasty tiny green French lentil, Le Puy, has a velvety texture and a spicy flavor. It's wonderful, along with an increasing number of heirloom varieties. My favorite way to eat lentils is sprouting them, thus enjoying their full nutritional value as part of live-food recipes.

Limes

In the mid-1700s, Scottish naval surgeon James Lind discovered that drinking the juice of limes and lemons prevented scurvy, the scourge of sailors on long voyages. Soon British ships carried ample stores of the fruits, earning their sailors the nickname "limey." It was later learned that vitamin C deficiency causes scurvy, and that limes are very high in this essential nutrient.

Like lemons, limes are useful as flavoring agents. However, unlike their yellow counterpart, limes don't impart a distinctive taste of their own when used as a cooking ingredient; instead, they tenderize and heighten the flavors of other foods.

Select brightly colored, smooth-skinned, heavy limes. Some may have small brown patches on their skin (russeting); this doesn't affect flavor. Don't purchase fruit that's hard or shriveled. You can store limes in the refrigerator for up to ten days. While lemons are harvested year-round, with slight seasonal peaks in May, June, and August, limes (also available throughout the year) are most plentiful from May through October.

There are many gadgets for juicing citrus fruit—including products onto which you press the fruit, reamers (my favorite) that you twist into the fruit—but it's simplest to halve the fruit and squeeze it in your hand, using your fingers to hold back the seeds. (Roll it firmly on the counter first to bring out more juice.) A large lemon will yield about three to four tablespoons of juice and two to three teaspoons of zest (grated rind); a large lime will provide two to three tablespoons of juice and one to two teaspoons of zest.

The juice of both the lemon and lime can be used instead of vinegar in salad dressings, and the acid in the citrus juices keeps fruits from browning; sprinkle some on cut-up bananas, apples, peaches, avocados, and other fruits to prevent discoloration. A wedge of lemon or lime, a squeeze of juice, or a sprinkling of zest freshens the flavor of many other foods. I use them many times each day.

Nutritionally, limes have all of the same benefits as lemons. Their juice has been applied to relieve the effects of stinging corals with good results. Less acidic than lemons, they exhibit a more pronounced action on the liver. They also contain furocoumarins, which make the skin less sensitive to light and help prevent severe sunburn—but don't use limes as a substitute for sunscreen!

And as if all of that weren't enough, a glass vase filled with limes and/or lemons makes for a dazzling centerpiece on your dining table.

Mango

Many Americans still consider the mango an exotic fruit, and it certainly isn't as popular in the United States as it is in the tropics. There, it's as widely consumed as the apple is in North America. The mango, which is one of my favorite fruits, tastes like a peach and pineapple mixed together, only sweeter. It's well worth the effort it takes to seed and peel because you'll savor every bite. It has smooth skin and orange-yellow flesh that, when ripe, is soft and exceptionally juicy.

Mangoes provide large amounts of the antioxidants vitamin C and beta-carotene, which can block the effects of harmful oxygen molecules called *free radicals,* which can damage healthy tissues throughout the body. One mango contains 50–83 percent of the RDA for beta-carotene and about 95 percent of the RDA for vitamin C.

It's not only antioxidants that make mangoes good for you; they're also high in fiber, with one fruit supplying almost six grams of fiber—more than you'd get in a cup of cooked oat bran. What's more, nearly half of the fiber in mangoes is the soluble kind. Countless studies have shown that getting more soluble fiber in the diet can help lower cholesterol and reduce the risk of heart disease, high blood pressure, and stroke. The insoluble fiber in mangoes is also important because it causes stools—and any harmful substances they contain—to move through the body more quickly. This means that eating more of this fruit can play a role in reducing the risk of colon cancer.

Select mangoes that are fresh, firm, and plump and have a pleasant, spicy aroma at the stem end. If there's no smell, the fruit will be flavorless. Ripen at room temperature in a brown bag until the flesh yields slightly to pressure, like a ripe avocado. As the mango ripens, the skin color intensifies (green-skinned mangoes excepted). Once ripe, the fruit may be refrigerated for several days.

Because imported mangoes are heat treated to kill fruit flies or pests, I select domestic ones, which usually come from Florida, California, or Hawaii. For a real treat, next time you make or buy salsa, add some diced mango.

Meyer Lemon

It was during my early childhood that I discovered this small, juicy, exquisite lemon. We had a prolific fruit-bearing tree in our backyard, and my mom put the juice into many of our meals. It was the most welcomed gift we gave to our neighbors. Prized for its amazingly sweet fragrance and flavor, the Meyer lemon combines the familiar qualities of a lemon with hints of orange and tangerine. However, it wasn't until the mid-1970s that every chef in California seemed to simultaneously discover it.

While I learned about them more than four decades ago, Meyer lemons actually had been growing in California, Texas, and Florida for almost 70 years. First hybridized in China some 400 years ago, they were discovered near Peking and introduced to America in 1908 by a U.S. Department of Agriculture botanist named Frank Meyer.

You'll find Meyer lemons with increasing frequency today in farmers markets and enterprising supermarkets. It's hard to miss them—their fairly smooth skins have a hint of orange mixed with yellow and a wonderful perfume you can detect when your nose is still a good several inches away. They're also very easy to grow at home in a temperate climate and can bear fruit year-round.

Use these fruits just as you would regular lemons: in dressings, marinades, sauces, or drinks or squeezed over grilled vegetables and other grilled foods. There's no better citrus to put in your filtered water, in my estimation, than the juice of a fresh Meyer lemon. They're also great for making lemonade.

Meyer lemons are high in vitamin C and contain alkalinizing and detoxifying properties. They're an exquisite lemon whose abundant juice has just a hint of sweetness. Whether using the zest or the juice, you'll find that they complement any dish.

Millet

The smallest of our familiar grains, millet is an ancient plant of Asia and North Africa and is gluten free (so it can't be used for raised breads). It's made into tasty flat breads and also can be used in pilaf or as a stuffing for vegetables. In the United States, millet is known principally as feed for birds and poultry. However, pearl millet, which is the major type grown for human consumption, can be found in health-food stores and some supermarkets, always hulled and usually in whole-grain form. The tiny, pale yellow or reddish orange beads can be cooked like any other grain. It's usually tolerated by people who are allergic to wheat.

Of all the true cereal grains, millet has the richest amino acid protein profile and the highest iron content. It's very rich in phosphorus and B vitamins. Due to its high alkaline ash content, it's also the easiest grain to digest. This unusual makeup allows it to be cooked without salt and yet be alkaline rather than acidic.

A cup of cooked millet contains nearly 110 mg of magnesium. According to research, eating magnesium-rich foods such as this grain (and tofu, avocados, spinach, bananas, and peanut butter) may help ease the irritability, sadness, and other emotional ups and downs that some women experience every month. Research has shown that women with premenstrual syndrome (PMS) often have low levels of magnesium. "A marginal magnesium deficiency could make certain women more susceptible to PMS," says Donald L. Rosenstein, M.D., chief of the psychiatry consultation-liaison service at the National Institutes of Health.

Millet is a good source of protein, which the body uses for building and repairing muscles, connective fibers, and other tissues. Getting more protein in your diet is particularly important when you've cut yourself, been burned, or had surgery. Without plenty of it, wound healing can be delayed. A cup of millet contains almost ten grams of protein. Compare that to a similar amount of brown rice, which supplies only five grams. While meat is also a potent source of this nutrient, it's also high in cholesterol-raising saturated fats. One cup of cooked millet (about 230 calories) provides as much protein as an ounce of beef and is low fat and cholesterol free, making it a superior choice.

Unlike brown rice, millet doesn't take forever to go from pot to plate, and it's very easy to make. In a saucepan, mix a cup of whole millet with 2½ cups of water; bring to a boil; then simmer and cook, covered, until the grains are tender, usually about 20–25 minutes. Fluff with a fork and serve immediately. Cooking millet in apple juice instead of water will add a bit of sweetness to the dish. For a creamier texture, stir frequently while cooking, which causes the grains to absorb more of the liquid.

You also can make your own freshly milled, nutritious flour from millet in the *Kitchen Mill*. (To order this excellent grinding mill, visit: **www.SusanSmithJones. com** and click on *Susan's Favorite Products,* then click on *Blendtec Home.*) I often make it because it lends a dry, delicate, cakelike crumb and a pale yellow color to baked goods. Fresh millet flour has a distinctive sweet flavor. When old, however, it's bitter and should be discarded. Millet flour is sold in natural-food stores, but since it turns rancid quite rapidly, it's best to grind it as needed. And because millet has no gluten, the flour should be combined with wheat flour for cookies, cakes, and bread. For sauces and some cookies and flat breads, it may be used alone.

Miso

Pronounced *MEE-so,* this delicious, all-purpose, high-protein seasoning has played a major role in Japanese culture and cuisine for centuries. It most often is made from a combination of soybeans, cultured grain, and sea salt by a unique fermentation process, which has been elevated to a state of fine craftsmanship in Japan. Unpasteurized miso is a living food containing natural digestive enzymes, lactobacillus, and other microorganisms that aid in the digestion of all foods and that have been shown to ward off and destroy harmful microorganisms, thereby creating a healthy digestive system.

An article published in the British *Journal of the National Cancer Institute* in June 2003 reported that breast-cancer risk was reduced by *one half* in Japanese women who ate *three or more* bowls of miso soup on an almost daily basis. Conducted by the Japan Public Health Study of Cancer and Cardiovascular Disease, the report monitored 21,852 women from 1990 to 2000. Postmenopausal women showed the highest reduction of risk. With high-quality miso available in the United States, we, too, can enjoy the protective health benefits of this miraculous food.

Since each teaspoonful of unpasteurized miso contains millions of active microorganisms that are beneficial to the dynamic digestion and assimilation of all foods, miso shouldn't be subjected to prolonged cooking or high heat. Add it at the end of cooking and turn the heat all the way down or remove the pot from the stove. I put a teaspoon in a mug or bowl and stir in hot water without any cooking. Miso soup should taste neither too salty nor too bland. The NATURE-FOOD should enhance the flavor of the soup but not overwhelm it. I also use this ingredient in dips, spreads, sauces, and salad dressings. My favorite miso can be ordered from: **www.southrivermiso.com.**

Papaya

Native to Central America, papayas now are grown in tropical climates around the world. On the outside, they look like yellow or orange avocados. On the inside, you'll find beautiful yellow-orange flesh that hints at the healing powers it holds. The seeds are edible, too; just rinse them and add to a salad for a nutty and slightly peppery taste.

One medium-size papaya supplies more than twice the adult RDA of vitamin C, almost 30 percent of the RDA of folate, and 25 percent of the RDA of potassium. They're also an excellent source of vitamins A and E and are rich in calcium, iron, and phosphorus. They're low in calories and, when ripe, contain about 8 percent sugar.

Like most yellow-orange fruits, papayas are packed with carotenoids, natural plant pigments that give many fruits and vegetables their beautiful hues. But these substances do much more than embellish a plate—they can save your life. The carotenoids in papayas are extremely powerful antioxidants. Studies have shown that people who eat the most carotenoid-rich foods like papayas have a significantly lower risk of dying from heart disease and cancer.

Papayas also contain *papain,* an enzyme that's similar to the digestive juice pepsin. Because this enzyme breaks down protein, papain extract from papayas is marketed as a meat tenderizer. Topical ointments containing the enzyme are sometimes applied to promote the shedding of dead tissue. (In "The Healing Power of Beautiful Skin" section, I describe two superb facial masks by Reviva that incorporate green papaya.) Papain causes the dermatitis that some people experience when handling papayas; this irritation isn't necessarily an allergic reaction.

A home remedy to reduce mosquito-bite irritation is to rub the bite with a piece of green papaya, its seeds, or a meat tenderizer made of papain. The papain digests or breaks down the irritating proteins injected by the insect. If you have allergic reactions to insect venom, do *not* use this kitchen remedy.

Although some varieties remain green when ripe, the skin of most papayas turns yellow or orange. Like avocados, they're lightly soft to the touch when ripe. If green, they'll ripen at room temperature. Once they've ripened, refrigerate them. Peak season is from January to April, but papayas can be found year-round.

Peppermint

In ancient Greece, people chewed a sprig of mint after feasts to settle the stomach, a tradition that evolved into our after-dinner mints. Peppermint leaves have been used to ease headaches and aid digestion for more than 2,000 years.

Today, peppermint oil is a key ingredient in decongestants and remedies for irritable bowel syndrome (IBS). In one study, people with IBS who took peppermint capsules were able to eliminate all or most of their symptoms. Peppermint tea is also effective.

In another study, German researchers gave 118 adults with persistent indigestion a standard drug (cisapride) or twice-daily capsules of enteric-coated peppermint oil (90 mg) and caraway oil (50 mg), another traditional stomach soother. (The enteric coating allows the capsules to survive stomach acid and release their oil in the small intestine, where nonheartburn indigestion develops.) After four weeks, the herbal blend was found to be just as effective as the drug.

Peppermint oil may elevate and open the sensory system, and its aromatic influences are purifying and stimulating to the conscious mind. In addition to volatile oil, mint also contains numerous biologically active constituents, including flavonoids (such as rutin), resins, tannin, and azulene. (If you use herbal oils, don't exceed the recommended dose, and keep them away from children.)

Mint of any kind is a balm for the entire digestive tract, regulating the stomach, liver, gallbladder, and intestines; it also regulates the sexual functions of both men and women. However, mint can just as easily stop periods, so it's best to be careful—and perhaps avoid peppermint—during the menstrual cycle. The deodorant properties of this herb have been capitalized on as well, and they make frequent appearances in mouthwashes and toothpastes to sweeten the breath.

If I get indigestion, I go to the garden, pick some peppermint, chew the leaves, and make tea. It works well for me. I often put one or two leaves of peppermint into my teas made of other herbs, especially those that are more medicinal and don't have the best aroma or taste. Don't give mint tea to children younger than two, as the menthol in it can make them choke.

You can use peppermint as an ingredient in recipes, but it can overwhelm more subtle flavors. The leaves are a tasty garnish for desserts made with chocolate or carob.

I keep a small bottle of essential oil of peppermint in my shower. As the water is warming up, I sprinkle a few drops on the shower floor and deeply breathe in the sensuous fragrance.

Pineapple

The pineapple is a symbol of hospitality and often appears in household-art motifs. Start noticing these images, and you'll soon see them on everything from brass door knockers to light fixtures.

A tropical fruit, the pineapple originated in Brazil, but most of the ones Americans eat come from Hawaii. The high sugar content and lush flavor make it one of the most popular fruits. Unlike most other fruits, pineapples don't ripen or sweeten after picking. Since they have no reserve of starch to be converted into sugar, they start to deteriorate instead. Look for large, plump, heavy fruit with fresh, deep green plumage. Skin coloring may be green or yellow-gold, depending on the variety. The base should be slightly soft, and there's generally a sweet but not fermented aroma. Avoid any that are old looking, dry, or starting to decay at the base. To ensure a uniformly sweet fruit, remove the leaves and stand the pineapple upside down at room temperature so the sweet juice concentrated at the base can run throughout. This NatureFood can be stored at room temperature if used within a few days. Cut into chunks, the fruit can be kept in a container in the refrigerator for four to five more days.

Pineapples are a veritable warehouse of valuable minerals and enzymes. One enzyme in particular, bromelain, is renowned for its health benefits. It helps digestion by breaking down protein into more easily digestible amino acids. In addition, it's also credited with reducing swelling due to arthritis, sports injuries, and trauma, as well as promoting the healing of wounds, soothing sore throats, treating laryngitis, relieving sinusitis, curbing appetite, and promoting the absorption of antibiotics.

As a cardiovascular support, bromelain also may help alleviate angina, help prevent and treat atherosclerosis, and inhibit the abnormal blood clotting that causes second heart attacks. Peroxidase, another enzyme found in pineapple, increases the production of cytokines, an immune-system component that stimulates cells to protect themselves against cancer.

I recommend pineapple to my clients to help detoxify the body and provide a natural diuretic. The fruit contains a fair amount of acids—notably citric, malic, and tartaric, which in their organic form exert a diuretic action, aid digestion and elimination, and help clear mucous waste from bronchial tissues. The citric and malic acids also improve the process of fat flushing. The greatest value of pineapple juice lies in its digestive power, as I mentioned, which closely resembles that of human gastric juices.

For one of the most delicious, nourishing smoothies, blend the following ingredients until you reach the desired consistency: pineapple, cranberries, a bunch of parsley, a couple of leaves of romaine lettuce, and a dash of cinnamon. It's always beneficial to add some greens into the mixture. If I'm out of parsley or romaine, I might add baby spinach, cucumber, or sunflower-seed sprouts. If I don't have cranberries, I'll add blueberries or raspberries. If I want to make it even more nutritious and delicious, I'll add some pomegranate or blueberry juice as a base.

Plums & Prunes

A cousin to the peach and the cherry, plums grow on every continent except Antarctica. There are *more than 140 varieties* of this colorful fruit sold fresh in the United States. They've long been prized as a quintessential food. In fact, so exceptional is their image that their name has become synonymous with desirability. Today, a "plum" job is a very attractive one. When it comes to nutrition, plums are pretty attractive, too. They're a good source of vitamin C and offer an excellent supply of other vitamins and minerals. And they really shine when it comes to ORAC testing. With a score of 949 units for 3⅓ ounces, they're among the top-ten fresh fruits. Of course, a lot of that antioxidant power comes from the purple pigments in their skins.

Prunes are dried plums, but not just any plums. The most common variety used for prunes is California French, also known as d'Agen. The transition from plum to prune is a carefully controlled process. The fruits are allowed to mature on the tree until they're fully ripe and have developed their maximum sweetness. Then, they're mechanically harvested and dried for 15–24 hours under closely monitored conditions of temperature and humidity. I've made my own prunes in my dehydrator, but it's really easier to purchase them, organically grown, at my local health-food store.

As with other dried fruits, the process concentrates the nutrients. Just 3½ ounces of prunes boasts a phenomenal 5,770 units for an ORAC score (more than six times the score for plums). Since antioxidants have been shown to slow aging, perhaps prunes should be added to the top of your grocery list as one of the star antiaging foods.

Prunes are a superb high-fiber food, too. Ounce for ounce, they contain more fiber than dried beans and most other fruits and vegetables. Over half of this fiber is the soluble type that studies have linked to lowered blood-cholesterol levels. But they're also rich in insoluble fiber, which is perhaps the key to preventing constipation. Since your body doesn't absorb this substance, it stays in the digestive tract. And because it's incredibly absorbent, it soaks up great amounts of water, making stools larger and easier to pass. Prunes also contain a natural sugar called *sorbitol* that absorbs water, adding another excellent bulking agent to get the intestinal plumbing working again. With their image problem—being known as the fruit that your grandparents ate and recommended to help provide "a moving experience"—maybe they should be called dried plums more often.

If you're not fond of dried plums, an excellent substitute is prune juice, which retains a far higher proportion of the whole fruit's nutrients than the juice made from most other fruits. The beverage is made by pulverizing dried prunes and dissolving them in hot water. Therefore, it still supplies fiber in conjunction with iron—3 mg per cup, or about 30 percent of the RDA, and 475 mg of potassium (14 percent of the RDA), about the same amount as eight pitted prunes. But it's also relatively high in calories—182 calories per cup of prune juice, compared to 110 calories in a cup of orange juice. To avoid excess calories, don't purchase brands with added sugar; prune juice is sweet enough on its own. Better yet, purchase organic dried plums at your local health-food store. Rehydrate them with purified water and then blend them (with the rehydrating liquid) and make your own delicious prune juice.

I usually plump the fruit overnight by placing the prunes in a heatproof bowl and adding boiling water to cover them. Cover the bowl and refrigerate until needed. You can drink the liquid as well as eat the prunes; the liquid will contain some of the sugars from the fruit. I also freeze cubes of prune juice as I do with pomegranate and other fruit juices and put a cube in my water and other juices or teas as a natural sweetener and nutrient provider.

Diced prunes, prune paste, and prune bits are used in prepared foods, particularly baked goods, to enhance taste and texture. Pitted prunes are ready to use directly from the package—but take it from me, be sure to check for the occasional pit anyway. The mechanical process isn't foolproof. You can find yourself with a chipped tooth from biting on a prune pit and making an emergency visit to your dentist for repair.

Pumpkin & Pumpkin Seeds

Just because Halloween only comes around once each year, that's no reason to forget about pumpkin the rest of the time. Fresh or canned, this colorful fruit (not a vegetable) can help keep you healthy for many months. Like melons, they're a member of the gourd family. They offer lots of beta-carotene (only carrots and sweet potatoes have more) and are the number one source of alpha-carotene, a cancer inhibitor that's even more powerful than beta-carotene. Researchers looking at the diets of more than 100,000 people found that those who consumed the most alpha-carotene had as much as a 63 percent lower incidence of lung cancer.

Carotenoids are deep orange-, yellow-, or red-colored, fat-soluble compounds that occur in a variety of plants. The compounds protect the plants from sun damage while helping them attract birds and insects for pollination. Carotenoids have been linked to a host of health-promoting and disease-fighting activities. They decrease the risk of various cancers, including those of the lung, colon, bladder, cervix, breast, and skin. In the landmark Nurses' Health Study, women with the highest concentrations of carotenes in their diets had the lowest risk of breast cancer. Carotenoids also play a major role in protecting the skin and eyes from the damaging effects of ultraviolet light.

Extremely high in fiber and low in calories, pumpkin offers other nutrients, including potassium, pantothenic acid, magnesium, and vitamins C and E. One ounce of pumpkin seeds provides 20 percent of the RDA for zinc, an important immunity-boosting mineral. And studies show that a compound in the seeds may help prevent benign prostate enlargement, a common problem for men over 50.

If you want to cook fresh pumpkin, look for those labeled "sweet" or "pie" pumpkins at the grocery store; the ones you carve are stringier and not as palatable. You can roast fresh pumpkin and eat it like winter squash; roast the seeds, too. Or peel, boil, or steam and then mash pumpkin flesh (or use canned pumpkin) for soups or breads. I also juice fresh pumpkins with some green vegetables and a few carrots for a delicious "carotenoid cocktail."

Pumpkin seeds are the largest and one of the most costly of all edible seeds. Often labeled *pepitas*—"little seeds" in Spanish—they can be scooped out of a fresh pumpkin and toasted. Remove the pulpy fibers; rinse the seeds in fresh water; air-dry them by letting them sit overnight; season to taste with a little olive oil, salt, tamari, or curry/chili powder; spread them in a nonstick pan; and roast in a preheated 350-degree oven for 15–20 minutes or until crisp. Cool completely and store in an airtight container in the refrigerator. I dry them in my dehydrator so they're still a live-food treat, full of enzymes.

You also can find these seeds raw in natural-food stores or order them through health-food catalogs. Raw pumpkin seeds are recommended by some to expel pinworms or other intestinal parasites. Considered medicinal for the liver, colon, spleen, and pancreas, pumpkin seeds are *tridoshic*, or balancing to all body types, when used in moderation.

These delicious seeds are rich in vitamins A and E, iron, potassium, magnesium, phosphorus, and zinc. They even contain calcium and some of the B vitamins. They're also a great plant-based source of omega-6 and omega-3 fatty acids. What's more, one ounce of seeds has as much protein—nine grams—as an ounce of meat. Of course, you don't want to eat too many pumpkin seeds, since about 73 percent of the calories come from fat (with 148 calories in one ounce of seeds) . But when you have a taste for a crunchy, highly nutritious snack, pumpkin seeds, in moderation, are an excellent choice.

Quinoa

Centuries ago, high in the Peruvian mountains, the Incas dined on quinoa (pronounced *KEEN-wah*). The name literally means the "mother grain." This ancient food isn't a true grain (neither are buckwheat and amaranth), but it looks like one and has similar uses. Recently, people living in the United States have "discovered" it.

Quinoa cooks quickly into a fluffy, delicately flavored dish that lends itself to many uses. It can be served as a substitute for rice, potatoes, and other starchy foods; combined with vegetables to make a pilaf; and added to soups and stews. While rice, wheat, and other grains are all prepared in similar ways, quinoa is smaller and more delicate and must be treated a little bit differently.

As quinoa grows, it develops a natural, protective coating called *saponin,* which sometimes has a bitter taste. To wash away the residue, rinse well before cooking. Because of its small, delicate texture, it cooks more quickly than other grains. To get the proper consistency, bring two cups of water to a boil, add one cup of well-rinsed quinoa, reduce the heat to low, and cook covered for 10–15 minutes, until the grains are tender and all the liquid has been absorbed. For variations, mix quinoa into your favorite rice-pudding recipe, or cook it in fruit juice or with dried fruits, then offer it for dessert or breakfast.

This NATUREFOOD is teeming with nutrients. One cup of cooked quinoa (made from ¼ cup dry) delivers *ten grams of protein* with an essential amino acid balance close to the ideal set by the Food and Agriculture Organization of the United Nations. The National Academy of Sciences calls it "one of the best sources of protein in the vegetable kingdom." It's particularly high in lysine, an amino acid missing in corn, wheat, and other grains. Lysine is important for helping tissues grow and repair themselves.

One cup provides about 4 mg of iron, more than any unfortified grain product. You'll also find other essential minerals, including 90 mg of magnesium, 175 mg of phosphorus, 315 mg of potassium, and 1.5 mg of zinc, as well as numerous

B vitamins, especially B$_6$, folate, niacin, and thiamine. Oh yes, let's not forget that you receive this panoply of nutritional wealth in just one cup, which has only 160 calories in the form of complex carbohydrates.

While most grains are good keepers, quinoa spoils quickly. To preserve nutrients and taste, it's best to buy quinoa only in small amounts and to store it in an airtight container in the refrigerator or another cool, dark place.

Sea Salt

For most Americans, dramatically reducing the amount of salt added to foods will bring health benefits. I limit my use of the mineral, and when a recipe calls for salt, I use only the very best—the Celtic Sea Salt brand. It's authentic whole salt from one of the most pristine coastal regions of France. Hand harvested and dried by the sun and wind, this product contains no anticaking or bleaching agents or other additives of any kind.

What's more, Celtic Sea Salt is highly recommended by many chefs. It's no surprise why. With a natural balance of minerals and trace elements, it's an important source of sodium chloride, which in small amounts is important for good health. Unlike ordinary table salts, this brand provides potassium, magnesium, and other important nutrients. (It also contains trace amounts of iodine, but not enough to meet dietary recommendations.)

This unique salt imparts a rich, exceptional flavor that enhances the taste of any dish. You can use it as a replacement for ordinary table salt in cooking, in baking, or at meals. In order to preserve optimal freshness and taste, Celtic Sea Salt is best stored in a glass, wood, or ceramic container with a loose-fitting lid.

As one of the most natural and healthful condiments, sea salt provides a wide range of minerals and trace elements that support the health of all bodily systems, including the immune, glandular, and nervous systems. Potassium, sodium, and chloride (all found in this item) are used to create electrolytes. Often called the spark of life, they facilitate the electrical activities of the human body, including the heartbeat, nerve impulses, and muscular contractions. They're also necessary for producing enzymes, which are responsible for breaking down food, absorbing nutrients, repairing muscles, and producing hormones.

Trace elements are also important for the optimal functioning of enzymes. My friend the late Bernard Jensen, D.C., stated that trace elements are valuable "spark plugs in the structure of enzymes and proteins." He also believed that trace elements help speed up chemical reactions in the body, protect against diseases, increase energy, and preserve youthfulness.

Many experts believe that minerals are more bioavailable when consumed as part of a whole-food complex. And some researchers, like Andrew Weil, M.D., believe that when minerals are fractionated and processed, they undergo a mutation that can result in many health problems. Sea salt provides a balanced mixture of vital nutrients, while enriching the taste of any dish.

Celtic Sea Salt brand is revered for its great taste and health-enhancing qualities. It's sold in thousands of natural-food stores throughout the United States and internationally, as well as through catalogs and on the Internet. It's available in three varieties, and I recommend that you get all of them. Light Grey Celtic, Fine Ground, and Flower of the Ocean will come in handy for all of your culinary needs. My favorite is the last—Flower of the Ocean. I can literally taste the difference and see the pink tint to it. It's the one I have on the dining table to sprinkle on top of my food before eating, if needed.

This brand of sea salt is certified at the source by Europe's Nature et Progrés to be free from contaminants; it also is certified kosher. Each salt harvest is carefully inspected, and the cream of the crop is hand selected to bear the name of the Celtic Sea Salt brand.

For more information or to order Celtic Sea Salt or a variety of other health-promoting products, please visit **www.celticseasalt.com** or call: (800) 867-7258. Also, ask for a copy of their newsletter, *A Grain of Salt;* their catalog; or *free* samples.

Squash

Based on ancient remains found in Mexican caves, we've been eating squash for at least 7,000 years. It was one of the nourishing "three sisters" in early Native American diets. (The other two were corn and beans.) These foods were considered so important that they were often buried with the dead in order to provide them with sustenance on their final journey.

After a few thousand years of relishing them, we now can praise their nutritional content, too. When researchers talk about the healing powers of squash, what they're usually referring to is winter squash, which is distinguished by its deep yellow and orange flesh. Pale summer squash, while low in calories and a decent source of fiber, is generally regarded as a nutritional lightweight, at least until future research proves otherwise.

Members of the same family as melons and cucumbers, all types of squash are gourds—fleshy fruits protected by a rind. In a nutshell, summer varieties provide some folate and vitamins A and C. Winter varieties are extremely rich in beta-carotene and are a good source of potassium and fiber.

The summer squashes include the chayote, pattypan, yellow crookneck, straight neck, and zucchini. The winter varieties include acorn, banana, buttercup, delicata (one of my favorites), dumpling, Hubbard, spaghetti, and turban. The flowers, immature and mature fruits, and seeds are all edible. The seeds can be dried and baked for a snack; they're an excellent source of iron, potassium, zinc, and other minerals. They also provide some protein, beta-carotene, and B vitamins. Squash boasts the phytonutrient alpha lipoic acid, which, among many other benefits, has been found to prevent wrinkles and premature aging (good news for baby boomers).

Winter squash is one of the best-keeping fresh foods. Uncut, it should keep for three months or longer in a cool, dry place; pumpkins will last for about one month. Winter squash that's stored has more carotene—and therefore more vitamin-A value—than freshly picked fruit. The same could be said for all carotene-containing foods, except that most deteriorate before the increase in carotene occurs.

Turnips

Part of the *Brassica* genus, the turnip is reported to have originated in Russia *and* Siberia *and* the Scandinavian Peninsula. (I'll let you decide.) Introduced into the New World by Jacques Cartier when he visited Canada in the 1500s, this vegetable flourished there and quickly spread southward. The Virginia colonists must have brought seeds with them; turnips are said to have grown there in the early 1600s. The Indians took to them at once, for they were superior to the wild roots they'd been eating. Indian women baked or roasted them whole in their skins, a method that brought out their full flavor.

A member of the cabbage family, the turnip has a round or top-shaped root; white skin with purplish or greenish crowns; and thin, green, hairy leaves. Often confused with its cousin the rutabaga, the turnip is smaller and more perishable; it also can be eaten raw and is most frequently sold with its tops. The two do taste somewhat similar, however, and are interchangeable in many recipes.

When shopping for turnips, look for smooth, firm roots with their root end and stem base intact. If these parts are trimmed away and the root is yellowed at the incision, the turnip will be lacking in flavor. Choose small or medium-small turnips, as large ones are often pithy and bland.

I love raw turnips; to me they have a refreshing, tangy flavor similar to mild radish, and they're pleasantly sweet when cooked. When fresh and young, they can be used raw in salads. Those grown during the hot summer months are often more pungent, but they mellow somewhat with cooking. When cooked with other foods, turnips have the remarkable ability to absorb flavors, making them succulent and rich.

Don't discard the turnip greens; they can be cooked in the same manner as spinach, slivered and stir-fried, or included in stews. The tops are generally found separate from the familiar roots. The mature turnip greens don't make good salad, as they're too bitter and tough. I juice the small, tender leaves to garner their nutritional value, but the stems are not used. Make sure that you don't cook this NatureFood in aluminum or iron pans, as these will discolor the roots and leaves.

One of my favorite ways to use turnip is grated raw in my salads. This serves as a digestive aid and even helps clean the teeth. Because of its sulfur content, it warms and purifies the body, while its alkalizing nature helps detoxify. Sliced, raw turnip is superior in terms of nutritional value, but cooked turnips also are a warming food and said to energize the stomach and intestines. If you have a weak digestive system, turnips may cause flatulence.

When my friends and clients come to me complaining about too much mucus or a catarrhal condition, I recommend juicing turnips and combining the liquid with some carrot, parsley, and lemon. It makes a tasty beverage that's really good for you.

All *Brassica* genus vegetables contain dithiolthiones, a group of compounds that has anticancer, antioxidant properties; indoles, substances that protect against breast and colon cancer; and sulfur, which has antibiotic and antiviral characteristics. This family of vegetables also mildly stimulates the liver and other tissues out of stagnancy.

Low in calories, the versatile turnip is a good source of potassium, phosphorus, folic acid, and vitamin C.

Wakame

Sea vegetables have been eaten in Asian cultures for centuries. Edible seaweeds also have gained a foothold in America and have steadily increased in popularity since the 1980s—no doubt due in large part to the rise in popularity of sushi restaurants. In the culinary world, wakame (classified as an edible brown seaweed, although it appears green) is known for its flavorful contribution to soups, simmered dishes, and salads. Seaweeds such as wakame are considered rich sources of protein, fiber, minerals, and vitamin C. This NatureFood's healthful profile has piqued the interest of the scientific community, with the sea vegetable being featured in several recent studies.

Animal research conducted at Mukogawa Women's University in Japan and published in *Clinical and Experimental Pharmacology and Physiology* in 2003 indicated that in spite of the high-salt diet, rats fed wakame had a higher resistance to stroke and an improved survival rate after stroke than animals in the control group. Researchers noted that a particular compound found in the seaweed, a carotenoid called fucoxanthin, probably contributed to this effect. When they conducted culture tests with fucoxanthin, the compound proved to be protective for brain cells.

Eating wakame also may improve heart health. In a 1999 report in *The Journal of Nutrition,* researchers at the National Institute of Fisheries Science in Yokohama, Japan, noted that wakame prevented high blood pressure in animals. Another study, which was published in a 2002 issue of the *Annals of Nutrition & Metabolism* by researchers at Tohoku University in Japan, found that an extract from this seaweed reduced systolic blood pressure and helped maintain the reduction over the seven-week study.

Mekabu, part of the wakame plant, also has been studied for its health benefits. The ingredient, which has a strong flavor that complements soups, appears to have an anticancer effect, according to research published in a 2003 issue of *In Vivo* by researchers at Japan's Kitasato University. Their investigation showed that mice given mekabu had longer survival rates in the face of cancer, and their immune systems had stronger reactions to the presence of disease. Research from Nagoya University School of Medicine printed in the *Japanese Journal of Cancer Research* in 2001 demonstrated that mekabu specifically suppressed mammary tumors in an animal model of breast cancer; and in vitro, the compound effectively suppressed three strains of human breast cancer cells.

If you want to take advantage of the healthful—and tasty—benefits of wakame, the only necessity is a nearby specialty-food store. Most edible seaweeds can be obtained year-round from gourmet shops, Asian markets, and natural-food stores. Many Asian and other cookbooks offer ideas for using sea vegetables in all kinds of dishes.

One of the ways I reap the benefits of wakame is to simply soak it in purified water and either drink the water or blend it with other vegetables for a wonderful, salubrious smoothie. With seaweeds earning the distinction of "the oldest plants on Earth," it's no wonder these nutritious algae have come to be featured in dishes across the globe.

Watercress

A spicy, leafy, vivid green from the mustard family, watercress is a wonderful addition to salads and fresh juices. Cultivated and wild watercress are the same variety, but the domesticated plant is generally larger—up to seven inches— and has a thicker stem. Choose bunches that look fresh and have no yellowed leaves. Very young cress is a light, bright green, but the knowledgeable prefer it "sunburnt"—that is, slightly older—when the leaves have acquired a delicate bronze. Wilted, bruised, or yellowing leaves are signs of inferior quality and improper handling. Wash with extra care, as the plant is prone to harbor aquatic insects.

Watercress is especially kind to the skin. If crushed and applied with a swab of cotton, it relieves irritations and helps heal acne, eczema, and other skin irritations and infections. Many herbalists claim that it's a good blood purifier. It contains the highest concentration of antioxidants of any vegetable, says Daniel Nadeau, M.D., medical director of the HealthReach Diabetes, Endocrine & Nutrition Center in New Hampshire, and co-author of *The Color Code*. Watercress is particularly high in vitamin A and calcium and also contains vitamin C, potassium, iron, magnesium, and traces of nearly all of the B vitamins.

Compounds in watercress appear to protect against cancer. When smokers consumed two ounces of the plant per day for three days, it spurred increased detoxification of nicotine, according to a clinical trial published in *Cancer Epidemiology, Biomarkers & Prevention* in 1999. And watercress is the number one source of an extremely potent anticancer substance called beta-phenylethyl isothiocyanate (PEITC). If you have high blood levels of PEITC, your body may be able to neutralize some carcinogens before they damage cells. In rat studies, the substance prevented tobacco-induced lung-cancer tumors from forming.

I enjoy the peppery and bitter taste of watercress in salads, juices, and vegetable smoothies. One of my favorite beverages includes watercress, romaine lettuce, spinach, bell pepper, cucumber, carrot, apple, lemon, and ginger. This refreshing drink is a great detoxifier, rejuvenator, energizer, and alkalizer.

As a salad green, watercress should be combined with lettuce (such as romaine) or other mild-tasting leaves. Or use it as a garnish, as an ingredient in soups, or in an avocado sandwich. It also tastes delicious in stuffings, omelettes, mashed potatoes, or cheese dishes. When steamed, it loses much of its bite and tastes unique. Add it to completed dishes, and use daily if possible.

Wheatgrass

A chlorophyll-rich, vibrant green leaf, wheatgrass is one of the most direct and highly concentrated forms of the sun's energy. When it's made into juice, it's an optimal energizer. Nutritionally, two ounces of wheatgrass juice is the equivalent to 2½ pounds of fresh vegetables and contains 103 vitamins and minerals. The juice is 70 percent chlorophyll and is very high in vitamins A, B complex, C, E, and K. It cleanses, purifies, and feeds the body and boosts the immune system. If you want to lose some weight, an ounce of wheatgrass juice each day will be very beneficial.

This NatureFood is also very alkalinizing to the bowel and soothing to ulcers, cuts, and abrasions of all kinds, both inside the body and out. It efficiently neutralizes the toxicity of sodium fluoride, which is used in the fluoridation of tap water (and as a rat poison). It may be taken internally, used as a wash for the throat and eyes, or as a topical application (scalp tonic and cleanser).

Cereal grasses offer unique digestive enzymes not available in such concentration in other foods—enzymes that help resolve indigestible and toxic substances in food. Also present are the antioxidant enzyme superoxide dismutase (SOD) and the special fraction P4D1, both of which slow cellular deterioration and mutation and are therefore useful in the treatment of degenerative disease and the reversal of aging.

People with allergies to wheat or other cereals are almost never allergic to them in their grass stage. The Champion is the perfect juicer to extract high-quality juice from the wheatgrass. I combine a variety of other vegetables (including some apple for a little extra sweetness), ginger, and lemon with the wheatgrass a few times weekly for that delicious, nutrient-dense tonic.

Yellow Split Peas

You are probably familiar with green split peas, since they're favored in the United States and Great Britain, but yellow split peas are the ones you should get to know. These split peas, which have a more pronounced nut-like flavor, are preferred in Scandinavian and other northern European countries. They're also commonly used in Indian dishes like dal.

Neither type requires presoaking, and both cook quickly. In addition to soups, they make wonderful side-dish purées. Whole dried peas are available in some areas; they work well in casseroles, since they hold their shape better than split peas.

Of all the legumes, yellow split peas have the most genistein, an isoflavone that may help reduce your chances of heart disease. In fact, they provide nearly twice as much of this substance as soybeans. They may protect against cardio-vascular disease by preventing clogging of arteries.

Genistein also acts like a very weak estrogen in the body. It competes with stronger, naturally occurring estrogens and in this way helps prevent hormone-dependent cancers such as those of the breast and prostate. This isoflavone binds to sites on cell membranes that normally would be inhabited by hormones that can stimulate the growth of tumors. In addition, genistein also can inhibit the activity of enzymes that encourage the growth of blood clots and tumors.

Just ½ cup of cooked yellow split peas provides nearly ¼ of your fiber requirements. Fiber may slow the release of blood sugar into your bloodstream, keeping your energy high. Store split peas (and all legumes) in well-sealed containers at a cool room temperature, and they should keep for up to a year. If left in a warm, humid environment, dry legumes will take longer to cook. Don't mix a new supply of split peas, beans, or lentils with older ones; the mixture will cook unevenly. And finally, store any leftover cooked legumes in tightly closed containers in the refrigerator, where they'll keep for three to four days.

PART V

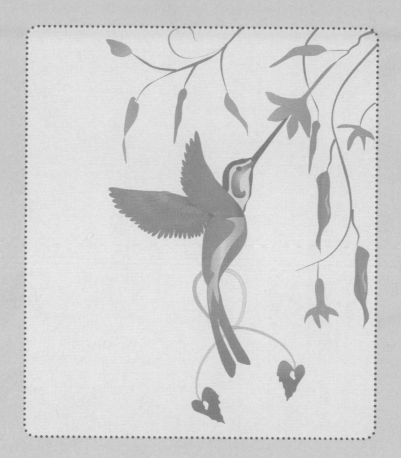

RADIANT HEALTH
AT A GLANCE

RADIANT HEALTH AT A GLANCE

NatureFoods keep you healthy in the following ways:

Abbreviations

MA	*mollifies arthritis*	BI	*boosts immunity*	BF	*improves brain function and memory*
PC	*prevents cancer*	EV	*enhances vision*		
HD	*staves off heart disease*	SA	*slows aging*	AR	*antioxidant-rich*
WL	*supports weight loss*	BS	*beautifies skin*	AD	*aphrodisiac*
		IA	*increases antioxidants*		

Radiant Health at a Glance Table

	MA	PC	HD	WL	BI	EV	SA	BS	IA	BF	AR	AD
Açai Berries	•	•	•	•	•	•	•	•	•	•	•	•
Aloe Vera	•		•	•	•		•	•		•		
Apricots		•	•	•		•	•	•	•			
Artichokes		•	•		•		•	•	•			
Arugula	•	•	•				•	•	•		•	•
Barley Grass	•	•	•	•	•	•	•	•	•	•	•	•
Berries	•	•	•	•	•	•	•	•	•	•	•	

	MA	PC	HD	WL	BI	EV	SA	BS	IA	BF	AR	AD
Burdock Root	•		•		•		•	•			•	•
Cabbage	•	•	•	•	•		•	•	•		•	
Cauliflower		•	•	•	•		•					
Cherimoya				•			•	•	•			•
Cherries	•	•	•				•	•	•	•		
Chicory	•	•	•	•	•		•	•			•	
Chlorella	•	•	•	•	•	•	•	•	•	•	•	•
Chlorophyll	•	•	•	•	•	•	•	•	•	•	•	•
Collards	•	•	•	•	•	•	•	•	•		•	
Corn		•			•			•				
Daikon	•	•		•	•		•				•	
Dandelion	•	•	•	•	•		•	•	•		•	
Dark Chocolate		•	•		•				•		•	•
Dates			•		•		•					
Evening Primrose	•		•	•	•		•	•			•	
Fennel			•	•			•	•	•			
Fermented Foods	•	•	•	•	•	•	•	•	•	•	•	•
Flower Blossoms				•			•	•				•
Go Green	•	•	•	•	•	•	•	•	•	•	•	•
Grapes & Raisins		•	•	•	•		•	•	•			
Green Beans			•	•			•		•			
Herbs & Spices	•	•	•	•	•	•	•	•	•	•	•	•
Jicama				•				•				
Lavender		•					•	•		•		•

	MA	PC	HD	WL	BI	EV	SA	BS	IA	BF	AR	AD
Lentils		•	•	•	•							
Limes				•				•	•			
Mango		•	•	•	•		•	•	•			
Meyer Lemon				•				•	•			
Millet	•		•		•						•	
Miso	•	•	•	•	•		•					
Papaya		•	•	•			•	•	•			
Peppermint				•	•					•		•
Pineapple	•	•		•	•			•	•		•	
Plums & Prunes			•		•		•	•	•			
Pumpkin & Pumpkin Seeds		•		•	•			•	•			
Quinoa			•		•			•				
Sea Salt	•		•		•		•				•	
Squash				•	•		•	•	•			
Turnips	•			•			•	•	•		•	
Wakame	•	•	•	•	•	•	•	•	•	•	•	
Watercress	•	•		•	•	•	•	•	•		•	
Wheatgrass	•	•	•	•	•	•	•	•	•	•	•	
Yellow Split Peas		•	•		•			•				

✳ ✱ ✳

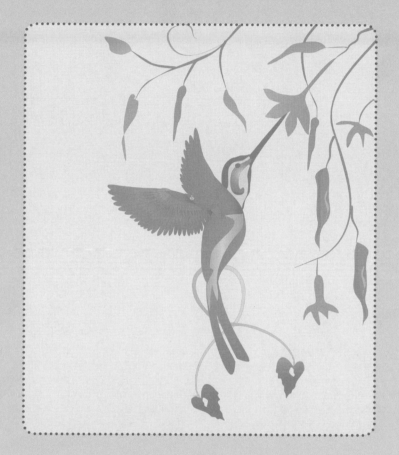

PART VI

Recipes

SALUBRIOUS
GREEN SMOOTHIE RECIPES

*"I look younger.
My skin is more supple now,
and I have fewer wrinkles than I did before eating raw."*

— CAROL ALT

As I've mentioned previously, *it's the little changes in your diet and lifestyle that make the big difference in the long run.* Adding easy-to-make, nutritious smoothies is a great place to start.

In the earlier section "Salubrious Green Smoothies," I recommended some of my favorite fruits and vegetables to use and offered a sampling of my most preferred and easiest-to-prepare recipes to consider. If you haven't read that section, you might want to peruse it now before you start experimenting with these recipes—and I do mean *experimenting.* You can't go wrong when you make smoothies; they're among the easiest and most delicious ways to ensure nutrient-bountiful meals.

Here are some suggestions you might want to try in your blending adventures. I encourage you to make at least one green smoothie every day and drink at least two cups. I usually average between two to four cups. Sometimes they're midmorning or midafternoon snacks, and sometimes they're my main meal, especially when I'm in a rush and don't have time to make much more than a delicious, nutritious smoothie.

For the recipes that follow, I combine a liquid base with about 50–60 percent fruit and 40–50 percent greens. To increase the nutritional benefit, I sometimes add other vegetables such as baby carrots, bell peppers, or sprouts. If you notice that your smoothie is too thick, just add more liquid; if it's not sweet enough, blend in a date or another sweetener suggested below. If it's not green enough, you can try a few more leaves of romaine lettuce or other leafy green. When possible, go for all raw (and organic) ingredients as another way to increase nutritional value.

The smoothie I make the most often combines pears, romaine or spinach (or both), water, and a dash of cinnamon. That's it! It takes about three to four minutes to make, including the cleanup of the blender.

I encourage you to become a smoothie culinary expert. Get your family involved, too. Kids love to make these and always enjoy the taste. It's such a great way to consume more greens without really tasting them. Enjoy!

Smoothie Ingredients

— **Leafy greens and other vegetables:** Romaine lettuce, red leaf, Bibb lettuce, spinach, collards, Swiss chard, kale, arugula, watercress, beet greens, butter leaf lettuce, sunflower-seed sprouts, or other wild or cultivated greens. Also try tomatoes, cucumbers, bell peppers, celery, fennel, squash, jicama, dandelion, burdock root, chicory, artichoke hearts, broccoli, beets, cabbage, cauliflower, corn, daikon, radish, sweet potato, yams, green onions, and sweet onions or shallots. Romaine lettuce leaves, especially the smallest ones, have the most neutral taste of all the leafy greens, and they add lots of nutritional value. I go through a head of romaine each day just for myself, and use it most often in my green smoothies.

— **Fruits:** Pears, apples, mangoes, blueberries, raspberries, cherimoya, grapes, apricots, strawberries, blackberries, cherries, cranberries, bananas, pineapple, papaya, lemons, limes, peaches, plums, nectarines, mulberries, kiwi, tangerines, persimmons, pomegranates, grapefruit, blood oranges, oranges, tangelos, and fresh figs.

— **Thickeners:** Ice; young coconut meat; fresh figs; bananas (fresh or frozen); soaked dried fruits such as apples, figs, dates, apricots, pineapple, cherries, papaya, and pears; nuts such as almonds, Brazil, macadamia, pecans, pine nuts, pistachio, walnuts, and cashews; raw nut butters such as almond, cashew, hazelnut, hemp, and macadamia; seeds (soaked and rinsed when appropriate) such as flax, chia, hemp, pumpkin, salba, sesame, and sunflower; oils such as almond, coconut, flaxseed, grape seed, hemp seed, and olive; miso—mellow yellow or mellow white work best with fruit combinations; and LäraBars. (All LäraBar flavors make great thickeners and sweeteners, and they are available at all natural-food stores.)

— **Liquids and juices:** Of course, this will vary depending on whether you're making fruit smoothies that include leafy greens such as romaine (which will still taste like fruit smoothies) or vegetable smoothies. Choose from any of the following liquids: purified water; freshly brewed teas such as peppermint, lavender, detox, açai, green, white, black, or literally hundreds of other individual or combination herbal teas; freshly made juices from your Champion Juicer; store-bought nutritious juices such as cranberry, cherry, raspberry, blueberry, kombucha, pomegranate, coconut water, mango nectar, and papaya nectar; hemp milk from Living Harvest; nut milks such as almond, cashew, macadamia, and walnut; and rice milk, oat milk, and banana milk.

— **Sweeteners:** LäraBars, pitted dates, bananas, date sugar, raw agave nectar, maple syrup, stevia (liquid or powder), raw honey, rice syrup, sucanat, and other natural sweeteners. I encourage you to refrain from adding any sweetener until the end of the blending since fruit is usually sweet enough alone. Also, start to reeducate your taste buds and get used to the natural sweetness of NatureFoods without adding extra sweeteners.

— **Flavor enhancers and supplements:** Black-cherry concentrate, tart-cherry concentrate, coconut, pure vanilla extract, raw dark-chocolate powder, and raw carob powder; edible essential oils such as cinnamon, ginger, fennel, and mint; flower essences such as orange blossoms, rose petals, and lavender; mixed dried fruits; cinnamon and nutmeg powders; BarleyMax, CarrotMax, and BeetMax; Sun Chlorella granules; E3Live; wheatgrass juice; Living Harvest Hemp Protein Powder and Nuts; Kyolic Garlic Liquid Extract; herbs such as oregano, rosemary, sage, and basil; ginger root; sea vegetables such as powdered dulse, kelp, and nori; lemon or lime zest; and even chili peppers, cayenne pepper, and hot sauce.

The Ultimate "Fast Food"—Salubrious Green Smoothies

The following delicious smoothies are quick and easy to make. All you have to do is put the ingredients into a high-quality blender (adjusting the amount of liquid, if necessary) and *blend!* After just a week or two of making these fabulous drinks (and the ones you dream up), you'll become a consummate smoothie aficionado and chef.

Ladies and gentlemen . . . "Start your blenders!"

Pear-Kale-Mint Smoothie

4 pears
4–5 kale leaves
½ bunch mint
¼ cup water

Place ingredients in a blender with some of the liquid. Blend, adding additional liquid if necessary.

Mango-Parsley Smoothie

2 large mangoes
1 bunch parsley
¼ cup water

Place ingredients in a blender with some of the liquid. Blend, adding additional liquid if necessary.

Peach-Spinach Smoothie

5–6 peaches
2 cups spinach leaves
¼ cup water

Place ingredients in a blender with some of the liquid. Blend, adding additional liquid if necessary.

Bosc Pear–Raspberry–Kale Smoothie

3 Bosc pears
½ cup raspberries
4–5 kale leaves
¼ cup water

Place ingredients in a blender with some of the liquid. Blend, adding additional liquid if necessary.

Blueberry-Celery-Romaine Smoothie

1 cup blueberries
1 stalk celery
4 romaine lettuce leaves
¼ cup water

Place ingredients in a blender with some of the liquid. Blend, adding additional liquid if necessary.

Apple–Berry–Sunflower-Seed Green Sprouts–Kale Smoothie

1 apple
¾ cup raspberries (or other berries)
1 cup sunflower-seed green sprouts
2 kale leaves
¼ cup water

Place ingredients in a blender with some of the liquid. Blend, adding additional liquid if necessary.

Mango Green Smoothie

1 cup fresh or frozen mango
1 cup fresh apple juice (or other liquid)
1 Tbsp. raw macadamia butter
2 Tbsp. flaxseed meal
4–5 romaine lettuce leaves

Place ingredients in a blender with some of the liquid. Blend, adding additional liquid if necessary.

Berry Green Smoothie

½ cup frozen raspberries
½ cup frozen blackberries
½ cup frozen strawberries
1 cup peppermint tea
1 tsp. organic lemon zest (rind)
2 tsp. flaxseed meal
5–6 romaine lettuce leaves or 2 cups baby leaf spinach

Place ingredients in a blender with some of the liquid. Blend, adding additional liquid if necessary.

*"There is absolutely no substitute for greens in the diet!
If you refuse to eat these 'sunlight energy' foods, you are depriving yourself,
to a large degree, of the very essence of life."*

— H. E. KIRSCHNER, M.D.

Sunshine Smoothie

1 cup frozen pineapple
1 frozen banana
1½ cups fresh orange or tangerine juice
½ cup fresh grapefruit juice
1½ cups torn kale leaves
3–4 romaine leaves
⅓ cup sunflower-seed sprouts (optional)

Place ingredients in a blender with some of the liquid. Blend, adding additional liquid if necessary.

Prune Green Smoothie

5 soaked prunes
¾ cup prune-soaking water
6 walnuts
2 tsp. flaxseed meal
½ banana
4 romaine lettuce leaves or 1 cup baby leaf spinach

Place ingredients in a blender with some of the liquid. Blend, adding additional liquid if necessary.

V-8 Green Smoothie

1 cup fresh carrot juice
½ cup fresh celery juice
3 baby carrots
1 tomato
1 green onion
1 tsp. Kyolic Garlic Liquid Extract
½ unwaxed cucumber
2 cups baby leaf spinach

3 romaine leaves
1 small red, yellow, or orange bell pepper
Dash of Celtic Sea Salt

Place ingredients in a blender with some of the liquid. Blend, adding additional liquid if necessary.

Persimmon Green Smoothie

1 ripe persimmon
¼ cup pumpkin seeds
2 soaked figs
½ cup fig-soaking water
½ banana
2 medjool dates, pitted
2 cups romaine lettuce leaves or Swiss chard (or other leafy green)
Enough extra liquid for the best consistency
Dash of cinnamon powder

Place ingredients in a blender with some of the liquid. Blend, adding additional liquid if necessary.

Apple Green Smoothie

1 cup apple slices
1 Tbsp. raw almond butter
1 Tbsp. raw hemp seed (Living Harvest brand)
¾ cup water or tea
1 cup leafy greens
¼ tsp. nutmeg powder

Place ingredients in a blender with some of the liquid. Blend, adding additional liquid if necessary.

Papaya Green Smoothie

1 cup fresh or frozen papaya
¼ cup raw aloe juice (Herbal Answers brand; see Aloe Vera in Part II)
¼ cup pineapple juice or papaya nectar
1 tsp. mellow white miso (or sweet miso of choice)
1½ cups leafy greens
Dash of cinnamon

Place ingredients in a blender with some of the liquid. Blend, adding additional liquid if necessary.

Fruity Green Smoothie

2 tomatoes
2 peaches, sliced and frozen
2 plums, sliced and frozen
½ unwaxed cucumber, diced
4–5 romaine lettuce leaves or other leafy greens
½ cup water or other liquid

Place ingredients in a blender with some of the liquid. Blend, adding additional liquid if necessary.

*"The doctor of the future will give no medicine,
but will interest his patients in the care of the human frame, in diet,
and in the cause and prevention of disease."*

— Thomas A. Edison

Citrus Green Smoothie

1 grapefruit, peeled and seeded
2 oranges (or tangerines), peeled and seeded
2 tomatoes
5–6 romaine lettuce leaves or other leafy greens
¼ tsp. cinnamon powder (optional)
½ cup water or other liquid

Place ingredients in a blender with some of the liquid. Blend, adding additional liquid if necessary.

Apricot-Plum Green Smoothie

3 large apricots
3 plums
6 romaine lettuce leaves or other leafy greens
1 tsp. lemon zest
1 cup water or other liquid
Dash of cinnamon powder

Place ingredients in a blender with some of the liquid. Blend, adding additional liquid if necessary.

"Nothing will benefit health and increase the changes
for survival of life on Earth
as the evolution to a vegetarian diet."

— Albert Einstein

Kiwi-Apricot Green Smoothie

3 kiwis
5 apricots
¾ cup unwaxed cucumber, sliced
2 sprigs parsley
2 kale leaves, spines removed
3 romaine leaves
1 Tbsp. flaxseed meal
1 tsp. lemon zest
1–2 medjool dates, pitted
2 cups water or tea

Place ingredients in a blender with some of the liquid. Blend, adding additional liquid if necessary.

Orange-Berry Green Smoothie

2 cups raspberries
1 cup strawberries
1 orange, peeled and seeded
6 romaine lettuce leaves
1 tsp. lemon zest
½ cup water or other liquid

Place ingredients in a blender with some of the liquid. Blend, adding additional liquid if necessary. With less water, it's a great chilled soup.

Blueberry Green Smoothie

2 cups blueberries
3 large kale leaves, spines removed
1¾ cups water or other liquid
2–3 medjool dates, pitted
¼ tsp. vanilla

Place ingredients in a blender with some of the liquid. Blend, adding additional liquid if necessary.

Raspberry Green Smoothie

2 cups raspberries
5 romaine lettuce leaves
2 medjool dates, pitted
1 cup water
1 tsp. lemon zest

Place ingredients in a blender with some of the liquid. Blend, adding additional liquid if necessary.

Detox Green Smoothie

1 grapefruit, peeled and seeded
1 orange, peeled and seeded
1 lemon, peeled and seeded
2 cloves garlic
1 Tbsp. hemp or flaxseed oil
1 tsp. fresh ginger, minced
¼ tsp. cinnamon
¼ tsp. (or more) cayenne pepper

Place ingredients in a blender with some of the liquid. Blend, adding additional liquid if necessary.

Peach-Berry Green Smoothie

1 cup berries of your choice, frozen
1 cup peaches, fresh or frozen
1 banana, fresh or frozen
2 cups leafy greens
15–20 almonds
2 tsp. flaxseed meal
¼ tsp. cinnamon
Pinch of fresh ginger root
Liquid of your choice

Place ingredients in a blender with some of the liquid. Blend, adding additional liquid if necessary.

Tropical Green Smoothie

1 cup pineapple chunks
2 mangoes, peeled and seeded
1 papaya, peeled and seeded
⅓ cup pineapple juice or papaya/mango nectar
2 cups leafy greens, chopped
½ cup sunflower-seed green sprouts (optional)

Place ingredients in a blender with some of the liquid. Blend, adding additional liquid if necessary.

*"I submit that scientists have not yet explored
the hidden possibilities of the innumerable seeds, leaves and fruit
for giving the fullest possible nutrition to mankind."*

— Mahatma Gandhi

Carrot-Apple Green Smoothie

1 cup fresh carrot juice
⅓ cup fresh celery (or fennel) juice
2 apples
1 Tbsp. raw cashew or almond butter
¼ tsp. vanilla extract
¼ tsp. minced ginger root
1 tsp. lemon zest
3 sprigs parsley
¼ cup cucumber
¼ cup basil
1½ cups leafy greens

Place ingredients in a blender with some of the liquid. Blend, adding additional liquid if necessary.

Coconut Green Smoothie

3 cups coconut water
1 cup young coconut meat
3 medjool dates, pitted
8–10 romaine lettuce leaves (or butter leaf)
1 sprig parsley
¼ tsp. vanilla extract
¼ lemon zest

Place ingredients in a blender with some of the liquid. Blend, adding additional liquid if necessary.

Purple Green Smoothie

1½ cups blackberries
1½ cups coconut water
3 medjool dates, pitted

1 banana
6–7 romaine, bibb, or butter lettuce leaves
¼ tsp. lemon zest

Place ingredients in a blender with some of the liquid. Blend, adding additional liquid if necessary.

Pink & Green Lemonade

2 cups water
1 cup fresh orange juice
½ cup lemon juice
½ cup strawberries
5–7 hearts of romaine lettuce leaves
¼ tsp. lemon zest

Place ingredients in a blender with some of the liquid. Blend, adding additional liquid if necessary. For limeade, replace the lemon juice and zest with lime.

Fresh Peachy Green Lemonade

3 lemons, peeled and seeded
½ cup raw agave (or raw honey), to taste
2 peaches, pitted
5–7 hearts of romaine lettuce leaves
4¼ cups water
Dash of cinnamon (optional)

Place ingredients in a blender with some of the liquid. Blend, adding additional liquid if necessary.

"Eat to live, don't live to eat . . . many dishes, many diseases."

— BENJAMIN FRANKLIN

Sunny's Luscious Sweet Green Smoothie

1 pear, cored
12 frozen fresh strawberries
2 bananas
1 lemon, peeled and seeded
1 medjool date, pitted
¼ cup apple juice or peppermint tea
¼ cup juice of blueberry, pomegranate, raspberry, açai, passion fruit, or combination
1 tsp. cherry concentrate (optional)
6–8 hearts of romaine lettuce leaves

Place ingredients in a blender with some of the liquid. Blend, adding additional liquid if necessary.

Fresh Fig–Kiwi Green Smoothie

4 cups water (or chamomile or peppermint tea), chilled
4 large fresh figs
2 large kiwi
3 cups romaine or hearts of romaine lettuce leaves
¼ tsp. cinnamon
1 tsp. lemon zest

Place ingredients in a blender with some of the liquid. Blend, adding additional liquid if necessary.

Nut-Nog Green Smoothie

4 cups almond milk (See recipes that follow.)
¼ cup medjool dates, pitted
3 bananas
10–12 hearts of romaine lettuce leaves
½ tsp. nutmeg

1 tsp. cinnamon
1 tsp. vanilla extract
⅛ tsp. turmeric

Place ingredients in a blender with some of the liquid. Blend, adding additional liquid if necessary.

Almond Nut Milk

1 cup almonds, germinated (soak for 6–8 hours, then rinse/drain)
3–4 cups water
1 Tbsp. raw agave or other sweetener (such as pitted dates)

Blend the almonds and water until the almonds are pulverized. If using a sweetener, add it during the last few seconds of blending. Strain through a cheesecloth or fine-mesh strainer and discard the solids. Refrigerate.

60-Second Almond Milk

2 Tbsp. raw almond butter
1 tsp. sweetener
1 cup water (more or less for desired thickness)
A couple of drops of vanilla extract (optional)

Place ingredients in a blender with some of the liquid. Blend, adding additional liquid if necessary.

*"He who distinguishes the true savor of his food can never be a glutton;
he who does not cannot be otherwise."*

— Henry David Thoreau

PART VII

❋ ❊ ❋

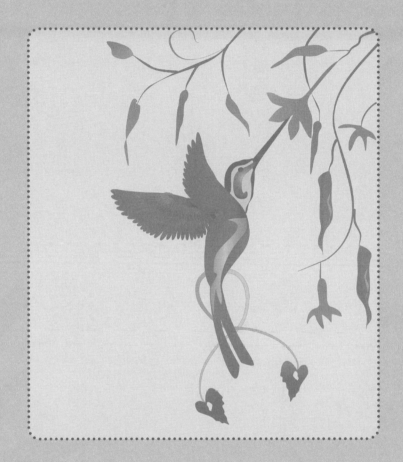

MOTIVATIONAL TOOLS

AFFIRMATIONS

"If you can dream it, you can do it."

— WALT DISNEY

For more than 30 years, I have been a proponent of using positive affirmations to keep motivated and create my best life. In conjunction with creative visualization, affirmations are a valuable tool you can use daily to help bring your dreams and goals to fruition. Most people underestimate the potency of their words. Always keep them sweet in case you have to eat them, as folk wisdom admonishes. Words, especially those with feeling, have power. Speak only ones that are loving, true, kind, and helpful. And always speak from your highest self, letting your words express the truth of your being.

Using affirmations is one of the great spiritual techniques of our time. These statements offer an opportunity to speak the truth about who you are and what you want to create. They encourage you to be true to your words and to your imagination. In time, you'll be doing more than just saying the right words, thinking the right thoughts, and visualizing your goals and dreams. Soon, you'll have adopted a whole new way of being. You will have aligned what you think, feel, say, and do.

Following are 40 affirmations you can use to get started. I also encourage you to make up your own, keeping them positive and in the present tense. Pick one to repeat softly out loud during the day. Repeat it silently as you go to sleep at night and again as you awaken in the morning so that your last thoughts before sleep and first thoughts upon waking are positive, uplifting, inspiring, and motivating.

In my books and audio programs *Be Healthy~Stay Balanced, Choose to Live Fully, Celebrate Life!, EveryDay Health—Pure & Simple,* and *Choose to Live Peacefully,* I offer more information on affirmations and how to use them effectively to change your health and life for the better. I also highly recommend the wonderful and practical books *I Can Do It: How to Use Affirmations to Change Your Life* and *The Present Moment: 365 Daily Affirmations,* both by Louise L. Hay. (See the "Recommended Reading" section.)

Affirm the Life You Want

1. I am open and receptive to a divine solution; I accept only the best for me.
2. God is working wonders in my life today.
3. I love and accept myself completely, as I am.
4. I eat foods that nourish my body and soul.
5. Small, nutritious meals are very satisfying to me.
6. My body is trim, fit, and beautifully shaped.
7. I weigh exactly what I desire, easily, effortlessly, and consistently.
8. I exercise vigorously on a regular basis, and I love it.
9. I give thanks for ever-increasing health, love, prosperity, and joy.
10. I always see the good in everyone and everything.
11. With integrity, I express myself easily and honestly.
12. I keep my word and make only those agreements that I can keep.
13. I am accountable and responsible for my own life.
14. I see problems only as opportunities.
15. I create relationships that are loving, supportive, and empowering.
16. Miracles are a natural occurrence in my life.
17. I am constantly giving away the very thing that I desire.
18. I deserve to be healthy, wealthy, and successful.
19. God is the source of my supply, and I accept only the best in my life.
20. With joy and thanksgiving, I salute and celebrate being alive.
21. With enthusiasm, I reach for the stars and accomplish the miraculous.
22. I live fully in my sacred partnership with the loving spirit within me.
23. I am alive, whole, and energetic.
24. Completely relaxed and confident, I rest in God's peaceful, supporting presence.

25. Each prayerful thought and act of kindness blesses the world with peace.

26. Giving and receiving generously, I am in the flow of good.

27. Nourished with divine wisdom, I anticipate and welcome good in my life.

28. A divine transformation is taking place, and a new me is emerging.

29. Uniting my imagination and faith, I soar creatively and abundantly.

30. God's grace fills my life with vibrant health, youthful vitality, and boundless energy.

31. Releasing the past and embracing forgiveness, I am refreshed, renewed, and revitalized.

32. In every area of my life, I am blessed beyond measure.

33. I make a positive difference in the world.

34. My body is a temple of divine life and energy.

35. I am healthy, happy, and enthusiastic about my life.

36. I am blessed in infinite ways.

37. I gratefully accept the abundance that is mine.

38. I have unlimited potential, and I accept only the best for myself.

39. I let go and let the spirit of love flow through me.

40. The light and love within me is inspiration and deep peace.

21-Day Agreement

"No man can sincerely help another
without also helping himself."

— Ralph Waldo Emerson

I, _____, commit that for 21 days, starting _____,

I will _____.

1. _____
2. _____
3. _____
4. _____
5. _____
6. _____
7. _____
8. _____
9. _____
10. _____
11. _____

12. _____

13. _____

14. _____

15. _____

16. _____

17. _____

18. _____

19. _____

20. _____

21. _____

_____   _____
Sign Here   Witnessed By (optional)

Make extra copies of this document and use it often as you make and follow through on your agreements with yourself.

After filling in the first sentence with your agreement, use the 21 lines to record a daily, "diary-like" progress report. For example, if you agree to walk every morning for 30 minutes, you write down what you did each day, along with a short commentary, such as the following:

1. Walked 30 minutes; legs felt strong and I'm motivated.

2. Still feel motivated, but harder to get up today.

3. I hate Susan. Her idea stinks. My thighs and butt are so sore today that I can hardly sit down. . . .

21. I feel so empowered because I kept my word and worked out for 21 days. I started because I demanded it of my body. Now my healthy lifestyle is my top priority, and I know I can do anything that I set my mind to do. Susan was right!

If you make one 21-day agreement each month, you will make at least 12 beneficial changes in your life each year. Whether you give up something unhealthful, such as any foods made with white sugar or white flour, or you add in something salubrious, such as drinking more water, eating more leafy greens, or exercising daily, at the end of 21 *consecutive* days (if you miss or ignore a day, you must start back over again from Day 1), you either will have established a new habit or will no longer crave what you gave up. (Please refer to the section called "10 Surefire Steps to Create an Abundantly Healthy Life" to learn more about the healing power and efficacy of making 21-day agreements.)

❋ ✻ ❋

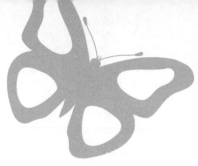

AFTERWORD

"Life is the sum of all your choices."

— ALBERT CAMUS

Close your eyes for a moment, breathe deeply, and ask yourself the following questions as you survey your body, mind, and spirit: *How am I feeling— physically, emotionally, and spiritually? Am I experiencing the joy of living? Am I feeling balanced? Or do I need a few last-minute reminders to take with me as I embrace and embark on life's great adventures today, this week, and this month?*

The core message of this book is threefold:

❋ You must earn your good health; it can't be bought.

❋ Get back to the basics; let nature do what it does best— keep you healthy.

❋ Live a balanced life; it's up to you to choose and create this for yourself.

Remember that in each moment you have the ability to awaken to your best self and life. From my extensive research and travels around the world, I've found that more and more people are interested in becoming truly healthy—not just physically, but also emotionally, mentally, and spiritually. (And if you are a baby boomer as I am, looking and feeling better are *very* desirable goals!)

Put simply, to be truly healthy, you have to do more than eat a colorful, whole-foods diet; jog around the block; and get enough shut-eye. You also need to be mentally and spiritually calm, focused, energized, and joyful. Making choices that integrate and heal body, mind, and spirit is what being empowered and living with balance is all about. Incorporating the principles I talk about in this book into your life will help you become healthier and happier than you've ever been! So here's a succinct description of those principles as closing guidance.

10 Steps to Balanced Living

1. **Exercise.** Develop a well-rounded fitness program that includes strength training, aerobics, and stretching. Make your regimen a top priority, and stay committed to it. Being fit is the key to enjoying life—it will unlock your mental power and physical stamina, as well as give you a positive outlook that will make each day a pleasure. Nothing does more good for you in terms of being vibrantly healthy, energetic, and youthful than a regular fitness routine.

As we age, we lose muscle, strength, bone density, and energy. Exercise combined with a living-foods diet is the best way to counteract that. Remember these three points: Move, lengthen, and strengthen. (For an easy-to-follow exercise program that produces results, refer to my audio program *Celebrate Life!* and my books *Choose to Live Fully* and *Be Healthy~Stay Balanced.*)

2. **Find time each day to be alone.** Enjoy the peace of your own company. By spending time alone, *especially outside in a natural setting,* breathing deeply and quieting your everyday thoughts, you can enhance your health, happiness, and peace of mind. Just 15 minutes of silence daily can nourish your soul. You may use that time to meditate. Notice how your mind is constantly chattering. Allow it to be still and open. Meditation establishes a quiet, dynamic mind.

3. **Express your feelings.** Not expressing anger or sadness can be extremely debilitating, especially if it's habitual. Beware of unreleased, uncomfortable emotions. Scientific studies have proven that people who don't express their feelings get sick more often, stay sick longer, and die sooner than expressive people. Repressed negative feelings feed on themselves; anger eventually may turn against the self and emerge as depression or severe anxiety.

Be aware of how sadness or fury affects your overall attitude. Just because you experience unhappiness doesn't mean you can't rise above it. We have the freedom to accept and embrace whatever thoughts we choose. Know that you can create your own dreams, no matter how difficult life can be at times.

4. Simplify life and slow down. Find joy in simple pleasures. Breathe deeply, smell the flowers, talk to the animals, sing with the birds, be with friends, greet the sun, scratch behind your kitty's ear, hug your dog, and make someone smile. Marvel at the miracle you are, tell people you love them, and laugh out loud—as often as possible!

5. Develop a sense of humor. A healthy degree of emotional detachment and hearty laughter can stimulate the immune system. Don't take things so seriously. Play more at this game of life, and be more concerned with your own integrity and experience than how you look to other people. Remember, angels fly because they take themselves lightly.

6. Cultivate the habit of gratitude. Be grateful for every aspect of your life—your ability to see, the food you eat, the air you breathe . . . the very fact that you're alive! Appreciation acts as a connecting link between you and every possible channel of goodness in your life. This attitude will help foster happiness and peace of mind and will help you live more gracefully and fully. Be thankful for everything that touches your path.

7. Graze. Eating smaller meals more often is good for muscle building and weight loss, and it even may be an effective way to reduce high cholesterol. When researchers from the University of Cambridge, England, assessed data on more than 14,600 men and women ages 45–75, they found that those who ate five to six times daily had the lowest LDL ("bad") cholesterol levels. Those who dined only once or twice daily had the highest, on average.

8. Become more childlike. Young children seem to know how to celebrate life. Be more flexible, practice forgiveness, and always leave time for spontaneity in your daily activities. Be less critical and judgmental. Let your inner child out to play.

9. Learn to live in the present. Don't compare what's happening now with what has gone before. Don't fret about tomorrow. Be fully present in each moment, freeing yourself from the past (which you can never regain) and the future. Look for beauty, miracles, and angelic guidance all around you every day, and celebrate the precious now. It is always the present moment, so learn to live in it fully. It's your moment of power.

10. Nourish your spirit. To maintain a healthy body, you also must nourish your spirit. The real epidemic in our culture is spiritual heart disease—low self-esteem combined with pervasive feelings of loneliness, isolation, and alienation. Many people who suffer from such malaise use food or stimulants such as drugs, caffeine, alcohol, sex, gambling, computer chat rooms, or overwork to numb the pain and get through the day.

Stretching, deep breathing, and meditation will relax your mind and create a greater sense of peace and well-being. When you're feeling balanced, you're better able to make diet, exercise, and other lifestyle choices that are life enhancing rather than self-destructive. Engage in physical activities that nourish your body and soul. One of my favorite pastimes is being outdoors and appreciating nature's beauty and magnificence. Some of my other cherished activities are in-line skating on the bike path along the beach in Santa Monica, California; gardening; or stretching outdoors.

Diet alone isn't enough if you want to achieve optimal health and happiness. Good nutrition combined with regular exercise is better. And when you combine these two with things such as being grateful, choosing peaceful thoughts, breathing deeply, and nourishing your spirit with activities like meditation and quiet walks in nature, you'll have assembled an unbeatable combination of good habits that will enable you to live with balance, reach your highest potential, and celebrate life to the fullest. (To participate in my telephone seminars on all of these subjects, please visit: **www.PagingSusan.com**.)

"Nothing in the world is more dangerous
than sincere ignorance and conscientious stupidity."

— MARTIN LUTHER KING, JR.

"If you want to get a clear picture of any condition in life,
don't try to see things with your nose on them! See them from the highest point,
from the plane of spirit, and you will be surprised at how different your problems look."

— WHITE EAGLE

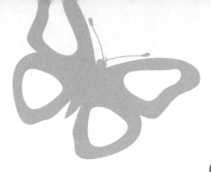

GRATITUDE

*"Life's most persistent and urgent question is
'What are you doing for others?'"*

— MARTIN LUTHER KING, JR.

I want to thank all of the terrific and supportive people who helped bring my vision for this book to fruition.

First, and foremost, this book wouldn't have been written without the loving encouragement of Louise L. Hay, my dear friend and kindred spirit in healthful living. As more and more people become as inspired and motivated as I have to live the way Louise urges us to, the world is becoming more vibrantly healthy, more loving, and more peaceful.

Special thanks to Reid for opening the door to my special series of book and audio programs; to Jill, my editor, dear friend, and earth angel who always guides my work with her gentle heart and sage vision; to Carina, my inspiring and tenacious publicist, who has been instrumental in filling my calendar with media interviews worldwide and bolstering my confidence when needed; to Donna and Mel, for always taking wonderful care of me; to Jessica, for being the wind beneath my wings and giving my words flight; to Summer and Diane, for helping spread my health message to millions; to Charles for designing book covers that are so delicious and resplendent you almost want to eat them (for the extra fiber); and to the entire Hay House staff, whose skill, expertise, and kindness is unsurpassed.

I also want to thank my dear friends Jim Lennon and Susan Taylor Lennon at Lennon Media, Inc., for their thoughtful suggestions during the creation of this book.

Finally, I extend my deepest gratitude to my cherished family members and extraordinary friends (you know who you are) for keeping this book in your prayers during the lengthy birthing process and for understanding those times when I needed silence and solitude during this writing adventure.

Thank you all for enriching my life.

❋ ❊ ❋

RESOURCES

RECOMMENDED READING & WEBSITES

"You must be the change you wish to see in the world."

— MAHATMA GANDHI

Alt, Carol. *The Raw 50*. New York: Clarkson Potter Publishers, 2007.

American Vegan Society. **www.americanvegan.org**

Barnard, Neal D., M.D. *Breaking the Food Seduction: The Hidden Reasons Behind Food Cravings—and 7 Steps to End Them Naturally*. New York: St. Martin's Press, 2003.

——— *Dr. Neal Barnard's Program for Reversing Diabetes*. Emmanus, PA: Rodale, 2007.

Baroody, Theodore A., Ph.D. *Alkalize or Die*. Waynesville: Holographic Health Press, 8th Printing, 2002.

Brownstein, David, M.D. *Salt Your Way to Health*. West Bloomfield, MI: Medical Alternatives Press, 2006.

Campbell, T. Colin, Ph.D., with Campbell, Thomas M., II. *The China Study: Startling Implications for Diet, Weight Loss and Long-Term Health*. Dallas: Benbella Books, 2005.

Cousens, Gabriel, M.D. *Conscious Eating*. Berkeley: North Atlantic Publishing, 2005.

——— *Spiritual Nutrition*. Berkeley: North Atlantic Publishing, 2005. (new edition)

Fuhrman, Joel, M.D. *Cholesterol Protection For Life*. Flemington, NJ: Gift of Health Press, 2006.

——— *Disease-Proof Your Child—Feeding Kids Right.* New York: St. Martin's Press, 2005.

Gianni, Kevin M., with Colameo, Annmarie. *The Busy Person's Fitness Solution.* Bethel, CT: A Better Life Press, 2007.

Good Medicine. **www.pcrm.org**

Hallelujah Acres Diet & Lifestyle. **www.hacres.com**

Hay, Louise L. *Heal Your Body.* Carlsbad, CA: Hay House, 2001.

——— *Meditations to Heal Your Life.* Carlsbad, CA: Hay House, 2002.

——— *Power Thoughts: 365 Daily Affirmations.* Carlsbad, CA: Hay House, 2005.

——— *The Present Moment: 365 Daily Affirmations.* Carlsbad, CA: Hay House, 2007.

——— *You Can Heal Your Life.* Carlsbad, CA: Hay House, 2003.

Health Science. The Journal of the National Health Association. **www.healthscience.org**

Heber, David, M.D., Ph.D. *What Color Is Your Diet?* New York: ReganBooks, 2001.

Hintze, Rebecca Linder. *Healing Your Family History.* Carlsbad, CA: Hay House, 2006.

Hocking, Melissa. *A Healing Initiation: Recognize the Healer Within.* Melbourne, Australia: Brolga Publishing, 2006.

Jacobson, Michael F., Ph.D., and the Staff of the Center for Science in the Public Interest. *Six Arguments for a Greener Diet.* Washington, D.C.: CSPI, 2006.

Jensen, Dr. Bernard. *Tissue Cleansing Through Bowel Management.* San Marcos: Bernard Jensen International, 2007.

Jones, Susan Smith, Ph.D. *BE HEALTHY~STAY BALANCED: 21 Simple Choices to Create More Joy & Less Stress.* Camarillo, CA: DeVorss & Company, 2008.

——— *Choose to Live Fully.* Camarillo, CA: DeVorss & Company, 2009.

——— *EVERYDAY HEALTH—Pure & Simple: Sure-Fire Tips to Heal Your Body, Restore Youthful Vitality & Renew Your Life.* CD Album. **www.SusanSmithJones.com, www.PagingSusan.com**

——— *The Healing Power of NATUREFOODS: 50 Revitalizing SuperFoods & Life-style Choices to Promote Vibrant Health.* Carlsbad, CA: Hay House, 2007.

——— *Recipes for HEALTH BLISS: Using NATUREFOODS to Rejuvenate Your Body & Life.* Carlsbad, CA: Hay House, 2009.

——— *Wired to Meditate, Celebrate Life!, Choose to Live Peacefully,* and other audio programs. **www.SusanSmithJones.com, www.PagingSusan.com**

Jones, Susan Smith, and Warren, Dianne. *Vegetable Soup/The Fruit Bowl.* Sarasota, FL: Oasis Publishing, 2006. **www.SusanSmithJones.com,**

www.PagingSusan.com

Joseph, James A., Ph.D.; Nadeau, Daniel A., M.D.; Underwood, Anne. *The Color Code*. New York: Hyperion, 2002.

Katz, Sandor Ellix. *Wild Fermentation*. White River Junction, VT: Chelsea Green Publishing, 2003.

Kenny, Mathew, and Melngailis, Sarma. *Raw Food/Real World*. New York: ReganBooks, 2005.

Khalsa, Dharma Singh, M.D. *Food as Medicine*. New York: Atria Books, 2003.

Klein, David. *Self Healing Colitis & Crohn's*. Sebastopol: Living Nutrition Publications, 2005.

LivingNutrition magazine. **www.livingnutrition.com**

Malkmus, George H. *God's Way to Ultimate Health*. Shelby: Hallelujah Acres Publishing, 20th Printing, 2004.

Marek, Denise. *CALM: A Proven Four-Step Process Designed Specifically for Women Who Worry*. Carlsbad, CA: Hay House, 2006.

Mars, Brigitte. *Rawsome!* North Bergen: Basic Health Publications, Laguna Beach, CA: 2004.

Meyerowitz, Steve. *The Organic Food Guide*. Guilford: The Globe Pequot Press, 2004.

——— *Power Juices Super Drinks*. New York: Kensington Books, 2000.

Moran, Victoria. *Fat, Broke & Lonely No More: Your Personal Solution to Overeating, Overspending, and Looking for Love in All the Wrong Places*. San Francisco: HarperOne, 2007.

Morin, Fléchelle. *Kissing or No Kissing: Whom Will You Save Your Kisses For?* Pacific Palisades, CA: Cheval Publishing, 2006.

National Health Association. **www.healthscience.org**

North American Vegetarian Society. **www.NAVS-online.org**

Nungesser, Charles; Nungesser, Coralanne; and Nungesser, George. *How We All Went Raw*. Mesa, AZ: In the Beginning Health Ministry, 2007.

Nutrition Action Health Letter. **www.cspi.org**

Onstad, Dianne. *Whole Foods Companion: A Guide for Adventurous Cooks, Curious Shoppers, and Lovers of Natural Foods*. White River Junction, VT: Chelsea Green Publishing, 2005.

Ornish, Dean, M.D. *Dr. Dean Ornish's Program for Reversing Heart Disease*. New York: Ballantine Books, 2005.

Pert, Candace, Ph.D., with Nancy Marriott. *Everything You Need to Know to Feel Go(o)d*. Carlsbad, CA: Hay House, 2007.

Pitchford, Paul. *Healing with Whole Foods.* Berkeley, CA: North Atlantic Books, 2002.

Pratt, Steven, M.D., and Matthews, Kathy. *SuperFoods Rx.* New York: Harper-Collins Publishers, 2004.

Reader's Digest. *Foods that Harm, Foods that Heal.* Pleasantville: Reader's Digest, 2004.

Rhio. *Hooked on Raw.* New York: Beso Entertainment, 2000.

Ritberger, Carol, Ph.D. *Managing People . . . What's Personality Got to Do with It?* Carlsbad, CA: Hay House, 2008.

Roizen, Michael, F., M.D., and Oz, Mehmet C., M.D. *You on a Diet: The Owner's Manual for Waist Management.* New York: Free Press, 2006.

Romer, Leslie Van, Dr. *Getting into Your Pants.* Charleston: Advantage, 2008.

Rose, Natalia. *The Raw Food Detox Diet.* New York: ReganBooks, 2005.

Schlosser, Eric, and Wilson, Charles. *Chew On This: Everything You Don't Want to Know about Fast Food.* New York: Houghton Mifflin Co., 2006.

——— *Fast Food Nation: The Dark Side of the All-American Meal.* New York: Harper Perennial, 2005.

Seidman, Michael D., M.D., FACS. *Save Your Hearing Now.* New York: Warner Wellness, 2006.

Shazzie. *Detox Your World.* UK: Rawcreation Limited, 2003.

Smith, Lendon H., M.D. *Happiness Is a Healthy Life.* New York: McGraw Hill, 1999.

Stoddard, Alexandra. *Happiness for Two.* New York: HarperCollins, 2008.

——— *You Are Your Choices.* New York: HarperCollins, 2007.

Tart-Jensen, Ellen. *Health is Your Birthright.* Berkeley, CA: Celestial Arts, 2006.

Thomas, Cathy. *Melissa's Great Book of Produce.* Hoboken, NJ: Wiley & Sons, Inc., 2006.

White Eagle. *The Quiet Mind.* UK: The White Eagle Publishing Trust, 1998.

Women's Healing Org International. **www.womenshealingorg.com**

Wood, Eve A., M.D. *10 Steps to Take Charge of Your Emotional Life.* Carlsbad, CA: Hay House, 2007.

Wood, Rebecca. *The New Whole Foods Encyclopedia.* New York: Penguin Books, 1999.

Yeager, Selene, and the Editors of *Prevention* Health Books. *The Doctors Book of Food Remedies.* Emmanus, PA: Rodale, 1998.

Yogananda, Paramahansa. *Living Fearlessly.* Los Angeles: Self-Realization Fellowship Publications, 2003.

RESOURCES

SOME OF MY FAVORITE
HEALTH-PROMOTING PRODUCTS

*"Be who you are and say what you feel because those who mind
don't matter and those who matter don't mind."*

— DR. SEUSS

I receive thousands of letters each year asking me to recommend some of my favorite products. Here are just a few that I wouldn't be without and that I recommend to everyone. Please contact each company for more information.

* Activated Air: **www.eng3corp.com**, (877) 571-9206

* Ancient Secrets Nasal Cleansing Pot: **www.ancient-secrets.com/ neti.cfm**, (877) 263-9456

* BarleyMax, BeetMax, CarrotJuiceMax, A Hallelujah Acres® Living Food: **www.hacres.com**, (800) 915-9355

* Bernard Jensen International for Dry Skin Brushes, Internal Cleansing Kits, Super Organic Rainbow Salad, and so much more: **www.bernardjensen.org**, (888) 743-1790, (760) 471-9977

* Body Slant by Age in Reverse: **www.ageeasy.com**, (888) Age-Easy

* Celtic Sea Salt, The Grain & Salt Society®, Home of Selina Naturally Products: **www.celticseasalt.com**, (800) 867-7258 (ask for free samples of their salt and learn about my favorite rebounder and other health-promoting products)

✳ Champion Juicer: **www.championjuicer.com**, (866) WE JUICE (935-8423)

✳ E3Live: **www.E3Live.com**, (888) 800-7070, (541) 273-2212

✳ Excalibur Food Dehydrator: **www.drying123.com**, (800) 875-4254

✳ Herbal Answers Aloe Vera Juice and Skin Gel: **www.herbalanswers. com**, (888) 256-3367

✳ Hydro Floss: **www.oralcaretech.com**, (800) 635-3594

✳ Ionizer Plus: **www.hightechhealth.com**, (800) 794-5355

✳ Kyolic Aged Garlic Extract: **www.kyolic.com**, (800) 421-2998 (ask for free samples)

✳ Reviva Skin Care Products: **www.revivalabs.com**, (800) 257-7774

✳ Spirolizer, one of my favorite, inexpensive kitchen gadgets that makes healthy food preparation a breeze: **www.livingnutrition.com/ healthshop.html**, (707) 827-3469.

✳ Sun Chlorella: **www.sunchlorellausa.com**, (800) 829-2828 (ask for free samples)

✳ Thermal Life Far Infrared Saunas: **www.hightechhealth.com**, (800) 794-5355, (303) 413-8500

✳ The Total Blender and Kitchen Mill: **www.SusanSmithJones.com**. Click on *Susan's Favorite Products,* then click on *The Total Blender* for more information.

> *"We must be willing to get rid of the life we've planned, so as to have the life that is waiting for us."*
>
> — Joseph Campbell

✳ ✳ ✳

RESOURCES

BOOKS & AUDIO PROGRAMS
BY SUSAN SMITH JONES

"As soon as you trust yourself,
you will know how to live."

— JOHANN WOLFGANG VON GOETHE

EVERYDAY HEALTH—*Pure & Simple (CD Audio Program)*
Sure-Fire Tips to Heal Your Body, Restore Youthful Vitality & Renew Your Life

This CD audio program takes the form of an encouraging and heartwarming interview with Susan and provides all of the tips and tools you need to achieve vibrant health; peaceful living; and an integrated life of spirit, mind, and body. Susan is a living example of the ancient wisdom, contemporary science, and 21st-century vision that she teaches. This CD touches on all of Susan's core teachings and explores the many facets that comprise living our best lives.

If you want to learn more about Susan—how she got started in holistic health; her passions; and her secrets to healing your body, looking younger, and bringing your highest vision to fruition—this is the perfect audio program for you. Susan is interviewed by radio personality Nick Lawrence, and together they'll uplift, inspire, motivate, and empower you to create your best life. Their engaging, conversational interview brings Susan's message to vibrant life and holds your attention from beginning to end.

In her gentle, loving, and efficacious way, Susan will teach you how to: deal with daily stresses with ease and grace; choose the best foods to heal your body; look and feel younger; lose weight; protect yourself from obesity, diabetes, heart disease, and many cancers; raise healthier children; release bad habits easily and effortlessly; understand the healing power of solitude, silence, and nature; reignite your self-esteem and find your purpose and passion; connect with your angelic helpers and Higher Power; and so much more!

Vegetable Soup/The Fruit Bowl

Vegetable Soup—The Nutritional ABC's and *The Fruit Bowl—A Contest Among the Fruit,* co-authored with Dianne Warren, are two picture books in one, teaching nutrition for young children. Via beautiful four-color illustrations and rhyming verse, the text introduces children to the connection between what they eat and how they look, feel, and perform. In addition to teaching about fresh whole foods—how they grow and why they are good—the book helps develop math and reading skills as children become active participants in the reading process. David Klein, publisher of *Living Nutrition,* praised it as "a wonderful children's book introducing the nutritional ABC's of whole foods!"

Choose to Live Peacefully—Book and Audio Book

In this celebrated book on CD, Susan examines the many facets that comprise a peaceful, balanced life, including how to take loving care of yourself, restore youthful vitality and create radiant health, connect with your inherent intuitive nature, and bring sacred spirituality into your daily life with ease and grace. In simple yet inspiring language, Susan offers an empowering 40-day, easy-to-follow program on how to live more fully—healthfully, joyfully, passionately, and peacefully.

Wired to Meditate—Audio Book

In this delightful book on tape, Susan shares her fresh, dynamic approach to unleashing your inner joy and developing your fullest potential. You'll learn how to use meditation and mind power to reduce stress and fulfill your dreams, neutralize negative emotions, make peace and prosperity your constant companions, release fear and awaken to your best self, harness your empowered inner presence to heal your body, practice simple breathing techniques that will lift your spirit and help you feel more serene, and much more.

Celebrate Life—Seven-Tape or CD Audio Program

From this enthralling and motivating series, you'll understand how to enrich and transform the quality of your life and experience greater health and more joy, peace, and love than ever before. Some of the topics covered include how to reverse the aging process; create a fit, healthy body; release bad habits; detoxify and rejuvenate your body; stay motivated to exercise; overcome stress, fatigue, and depression; build loving, supportive relationships; and live more from inner guidance. This set includes seven motivational presentations, six guided meditations, and a flyer with Susan's favorite positive affirmations to guide you on creating the life you desire and deserve.

Live Recordings

The following two-tape albums were recorded live at Susan's popular series of Healthy Living seminars presented worldwide.

* ❋ *Choose to Live a Balanced Life:* How to Be Healthy, Live Peacefully & Celebrate Life

* ❋ *Make Your Life a Great Adventure:* Living an Ordinary Life in an Extraordinary Way

* ❋ *A Fresh Start:* Rejuvenate Your Body and Life Each & Every Day

❦ ❦ ❦

To order all of Susan's books and audio programs, visit: **www.SusanSmithJones. com, www.PagingSusan.com; 800-843-5743**, Monday to Friday, 9 A.M. to 4 P.M. PT.

❋ ❋ ❋

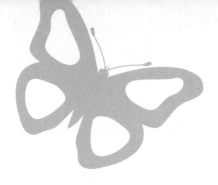

INDEX

21-day agreement, 15, 203–5

Academy of Otolaryngology, 84
açai berries, 37–39
    ORAC test and, 38
accountability, 16
Activated Air, 80–81
affirmations, 199–201
Agarwal, Rajesh, 43
aging, premature
    açai berries and, 38–39
    antioxidants and, 34, 38
    barley grass and, 45
    blueberries and, 47–48
    cherries and, 53–54
    plums, prunes and, 159
    sleep and, 91–92
    See also Radiant Health at
      a Glance Table

Airola, Paavo: *Health Secrets From
    Europe,* 111
aloe vera, 39–41
alpha lipoic acid, 59
    squash and, 165
Alt, Carol, 179
American Journal of Clinical Nutrition, 64
Ancient Secrets Nasal Cleansing Pot, 88
animal testing, 11
Annals of Nutrition & Metabolism, 167
antioxidants, 43, 59
    açai berries and, 37
    aging, premature and, 34, 38
    apricots and, 41
    cancer and, 43, 47
    chocolate and, 64
    collards and, 59
    fermented foods and, 71
    ORAC test and, 37

papayas and, 156
plums, prunes and, 159
See also bioflavonoids; Radiant
        Health at a Glance Table
Aphanizomenom flos-aquae (AFA), 141
aphrodisiac properties
    arugula and, 44
    burdock root and, 49
    cherimoya and, 52
    See also Radiant Health at
        a Glance Table
apricots, 41–42
arthritis, xx
    açai berries and, 38
    burdock root and, 49
    cherries and, 54
    evening primrose and, 66–68
    green vegetables and, 140
    See also Radiant Health at
        a Glance Table
Arthritis Foundation, 54
artichokes, 42–44
arugula, 44
"as if" acting, 17–18

baby boomers, 8
balanced living, 207
    10 steps for, 208–10
barley grass, 44–46
BarleyMax, 45–46
Barnard, Neal, i
basics, back to, 207
basil, 145
BE HEALTHY~STAY BALANCED (Jones), 12, 15,
        18, 25, 58, 93–94, 99, 200, 208
Belsinger, Susan: *Flowers in the Kitchen,* 72
berries, 46–48
    ORAC test and, 46
beta-carotene, 41

apricots and, 41
arugula and, 44
chicory and, 55
collards and, 58–59
mangoes and, 152
pumpkins and, 160–61
beta-phenylethyl isothiocyanate
        (PEITC), 168
bioflavonoids, 35, 45
    cauliflower and, 51
    grapes and, 142
blackberries, 48
Blendtec
    Kitchen Mill, 154
    The Total Blender, 131
blood pressure, elevated
    açai berries and, 38–39
    evening primrose and, 67
    grapes and, 142
    green vegetables and, 140
    lentils and, 150
blueberries, 47–48
bok choy, 50
brain function and memory, 8, 93
    alpha lipoic acid and, 59
    ORAC test and, 38
    sleep and, 91
    See also Radiant Health at
        a Glance Table
breathing
    diaphragm and, 78–79
    harmony and rhythm and, 79–80
    stress and, 77–78
    thorax and, 78
British Journal of Nutrition, 55
broccoli, 51, 56
bromelain, 158
burdock root, 48–49
"Butterfly and the Skater, The," 127–28

B vitamins
    cherimoya and, 53
    E3Live and, 141
    fermented foods and, 71
    millet and, 153
cabbage, 49–51
Camus, Albert, 207
cancer
    artichokes and, 42–43
    cabbage and, 49–50
    cauliflower and, 51–52
    cherries and, 53–54
    chicory and, 55
    chlorophyll and, 57–58
    collards and, 59
    corn and, 60–61
    daikon and, 61
    dark chocolate and, 63–64
    grapes and, 142
    green vegetables and, 140
    lavender and, 149
    miso and, 155
    papayas and, 156
    pineapple and, 158
    pumpkins and, 160–61
    turmeric and, 147–48
    wakame and, 167
    watercress and, 168
    See also Radiant Health at
        a Glance Table
Cancer, 39
*Cancer Epidemiology, Biomarkers &
    Prevention,* 168
Cancer Letter, 64
Captain Cook, 69
Cartier, Jacques, 165–66
cataracts, 41
cauliflower, 51–52
Celebrate Life! (Jones), 208

Celtic Sea Salt, 70, 163–64
    rebounder, 120
Champion 2000+ Juicer, 131–32
Chan, Tolentin, ii
cherimoya, 52–53
cherries, 53–54
chicory, 55
children, life celebration and, 209
chlorella, 55–57, 141
Chlorella (Jensen), 55–56
chlorophyll, 57–58, 140–41
    wheatgrass and, 169
Chocolate-Sweet Potato Smoothie, 64
choices, food and, 21
cholesterol, 41
    açai berries and, 38
    artichokes and, 42
    cranberries and, 47
    dark chocolate and, 64
    evening primrose and, 67–68
    fermented foods and, 71
    grapes, raisins and, 142
    grazing and, 209
    lentils and, 150
    mangoes and, 152
    millet and, 154
    plant-based diet and, 35
    prostaglandin E1 series and, 67
    prunes and, 159
Choose to Live Fully (Jones), 12, 15, 18,
    93, 200, 208
Choose to Live Peacefully (Jones), 12, 18,
    93, 102, 200
cinnamon, 144–46
*Clinical and Experimental Pharmacology
    and Physiology,* 167
collards, 58–59
Color Code (Nadeau), 168
Columbia University, 28–29

Committee on Environmental
    Quality, 121
Conscious Eating (Cousens), 141
constipation
    plums, prunes and, 159
    tarragon and, 146
Cook, Chuck, ii
Cook, Denise, ii
corn, 59–61
cortisol, 99, 101
    sleep and, 91
Courage to Be (Tillich), 123
Cousens, Gabriel, iii
    Conscious Eating, 141
Cousins, Norman, 19
criticism and judgments, letting go of, 18
Culpeper, Nicholas, 68
custard apple. *See* cherimoya
daikon, 61–62
dandelion, 62–63
Danielle case study, 25–28
dark chocolate, 63–64
dates, 65–66
decorative flowers, 72
DeGeneres, Ellen, 231
Dement, William C.: *Promise of Sleep,* 92
Department of Agriculture (USDA)
    food pyramid, 130
depression, 19, 33
    gamma-linoleic acid (GLA) and, 67
    lavendar and, 149
    rosemary and, 147
    sleep and, 91
Detox Your World (Shazzie), 107
diabetes, xx
    basil and, 145
    cinnamon and, 145
    dandelion and, 63
    green beans and, 144

lentils and, 150
Dickinson, Emily, 103
diet
    breast cancer and, 34
    diabetes and, 34
    fresh produce and, 129–30
    kidney stones and, 34
    mental performance and, 34
    nutrients and, 22–23
    prostate cancer and, 34
    See also specific NATUREFOODS
digestion
    açai berries and, 37
    aloe vera and, 39
    burdock root and, 49
    cabbage and, 50
    chicory and, 55
    daikon and, 61
    peppermint and, 156–57
    pineapple and, 158
    plums, prunes and, 159–60
    wheatgrass and, 169
discipline and commitment, 15
Disney, Walt, 199
diuretics, 63
    daikon as, 61
    dandelion as, 63
    green beans as, 144
    pineapple as, 158
    rosemary as, 147
Drapeau, Christian: *Primordial Food
    Aphanizomenon flos-aquae,* 141
Duke, James, 147
DYNO-Mill, 56

E3Live, 141–42
    B vitamins and, 141
eating disorders, 95–96
Edison, Thomas A., 187

Einstein, Albert, 188
ellagic acid, 142
Emerson, Ralph Waldo, 7, 89, 203
endorphins, 18–19
Euripides, 21
evening primrose, 66–68
    Barlean's evening-primrose oil, 68
EveryDay Health—Pure & Simple, 12, 93, 200
Excalibur food dehydrator, 143, 218
exercise programs, 208
    101 reasons for, 117–20
    higher intensity bursts and, 98–99
    mental factors and, 13–14
    metabolism and, 98
    Surefire Steps and, 14–15
fat loss steps, 97–102
    See also weight loss
feelings, expression of, 208–9
fennel, 68–69, 146
fermented foods, 69–71
    scurvy and, 69–70
fever, saunas and, 114
fiber, 36, 167
    açai berries and, 37
    artichokes and, 42
    cauliflower and, 51
    cherimoyas and, 53
    corn and, 60
    dates and, 65
    fennel and, 69
    jicama and, 148
    lentils and, 150
    mangoes and, 152
    prunes and, 159–60
    pumpkins and, 161
    raisins and, 143
    squash and, 164–65
    wakame and, 167

    yellow split peas and, 170
Finland, 111–12
flower blossoms, 71–73
Flowers in the Kitchen (Belsinger), 72
Franklin, Benjamin, 95, 193
Frawley, David: *Neti,* 87
free radicals
    artichokes and, 43
    barley grass and, 45
    berries and, 47
    cherries and, 53–54
French tarragon, 146
fruit blossoms, 72
Fuhrman, Joel, i

gamma-linoleic acid (GLA)
    aloe vera and, 40
    evening primrose and, 67
Gandhi, Mahatma, 191, 213
Gattefossé, René-Maurice, 149–50
genistein, 35, 170
Goethe, Johann Wolfgang von, 219
Goldstein, Allan L., 45
Grain of Salt, A (Celtic), 164
grapes, 142–43
gratitude and appreciation, 17, 209
grazing, 209
green beans, 143–44
green foods, health and, 58
Grudnik, Lynn, iii

Hallelujah Acres, 46
Hallelujah Acres Diet and Lifestyle, 71
Hay, Louise L., 13, 231
    I Can Do It, 200
    Present Moment, 200
Healing Power of NatureFoods (Jones), 7, 25, 36, 58, 64, 94, 99

health
    diet and, 33–34
    earning, 207
    lifestyle changes and, 33
    mental factors and, 11, 13
    NatureFoods and, 11–12
    physical factors and, 11
    plant-based diet and, 35–36
    spending and, 10–11
    See also specific illnesses and conditions
Health Secrets From Europe (Airola), 111
heart disease
    apricots and, 41
    artichokes and, 42
    berries and, 47
    corn and, 60–61
    dark chocolate and, 63–64
    evening primrose and, 67
    grapes and, 142
    green vegetables and, 140
    lentils and, 150
    pineapple and, 158
    wakame and, 167
    See also Radiant Health at a Glance Table
Herbal Force, 41
herb blossoms, 72
Herbes de Provence, 149
Heyman, Jeri L., 40–41
High Tech Health, 115
Hippocrates, 7, 68
human body
    adaptations and, 22–23
    diet, nutrients and, 9–10
    loving care of, 16–17
    positive changes to, 9–10
    self-worth and, 8
humor, sense of, 209

Hydro Floss, 65

I Can Do It (Hay), 200
Idol, Olin, ii
immunity, boosting, 25, 36
    pumpkins and, 161
    See also Radiant Health at a Glance Table
India, 68
Industrial Medicine and Surgery, 39
infections
    açai berries and, 39
    apricots and, 41
    daikon and, 61
    fermented foods and, 71
    oregano and, 146
    saunas and, 113
    watercress and, 168
Internal Cleanse Tool Kit, 109
International Journal of Dermatology, 39
irritable bowel syndrome (IBS), peppermint and, 156–57

Japanese Journal of Cancer Research, 167
Jensen, Bernard, 163–64
    Chlorella, 55–56
jicama, 148
Jones, Susan Smith, contact information for, vi, 94, 102, 210, 221, 230
Journal of Nutrition, 167
Journal of Pharmaceutical Sciences, 39
Journal of the American Medical Association, 64
Journal of the National Cancer Institute, 155
Katz, Ellix: *Wild Fermentation,* 70
Khachik, Frederick, 41
King, Martin Luther, Jr., 210, 211
Kirschner, H. E., 184

kombucha, 71, 133
kvass, 71

laughter, 18–19
lavender, 149–50
Lawrence, Nick, iv
lentils, 150
limes, 151
Lind, James, 151
Living Harvest, 133
Lotus Brands, Inc., 88
loving changes, 22
loving thoughts, 19
lycopene, 35, 41
lysine, 162

macronutrients versus micronutrients,
    45, 47
magnesium
    diet and, 154
    millet and, 154
    premenstrual syndrome (PMS)
        and, 154
mangoes, 152
Marx Brothers, 19
May, Paul, 57
meditation, 101–2, 208, 210
    nutrition and, 24
    positive attitude and, 106
melatonin, 53–54
    sleep and, 93
menstruation, peppermint and, 157
metabolism
    grazing and, 99
    muscle mass and, 97–98
    resistance training and, 97–98
    water, drinking of and, 99–100
methyl hydroxy chalcone polymer
    (MHCP), 145

Meyer, Frank, 153
Meyer lemons, 152–53
Michnovicz, Jon, 49–50
millet, 153–54
miso, 70, 155
Monroe, Marilyn, 42
Moore, Thomas, 21
mucus, 62
    neti and, 85–86
    sedentary lifestyle and, 85
    turnips and, 166
Mukhtar, Hasan, 43

Nadeau, Daniel: *Color Code*, 168
National Academy of Sciences, 162
Nature, 64
NatureFoods, 3, 36–37
    health and, 11–12
    See also specific foods
neti, 83–88
    benefits of, 87
    yoga and, 84
Neti (Frawley), 87
noise, 121–22
nutrition
    cultural and commercial
        conditioning and, 23
    eating process and, 24
    immediate gratification and, 23
    meditation and, 24
    senses, retraining of, and, 24
obesity, 35, 95–96
    green vegetables and, 140
omega-3 fatty acids, 100
    flaxseed meal and, 133
    pumpkins and, 161–62
ORAC. *See* Oxygen Radical Absorbance
    Capacity (ORAC)
Oral Surgery, 39

oregano, 146

Organic Hemp Protein, 133

Organization for Economic Cooperation and Development (OECD), 140

Oxygen Radical Absorbance Capacity (ORAC), 37–38

    fruits and, 46

    plums and prunes and, 159

PagingSusan.com, vi, 94, 102, 210, 221

Pagnol, Marcel, 149

papain, 156

papayas, 155–56

Paracelsus, 73

Paramahansa Yogananda, 83

peppermint, 156–57

perillyl alcohol, 53

phenols, 47

pineapple, 157–58

Plato, 17

plums, 159

premenstrual syndrome (PMS), 154

present, living in the, 209–10

Present Moment (Hay), 200

Preuss, Harry G., 146

Prevention, 54

Primordial Food Aphanizomenon flos-aquae (Drapeau), 141

products, health-promoting, 217–18

Promise of Sleep (Dement), 92

prostaglandin E1 series, 67

pumpkins, 160–62

    seeds of, 161

Pythagoras, 24, 117

quercetin, 54, 142

Quiet Mind (White Eagle), 123

quinoa, 162–63

Radiant Health at a Glance Table, 173–75

raisins, 143

Ray, Lisa, iii

RDA. *See* Recommended Daily Allowance (RDA)

rebounder, 120, 217

recipes. *See under* smoothies, salubrious

Recipes for HEALTH BLISS, 25, 58, 99

Recommended Daily Allowance (RDA), 37

    See also specific foods and substances

Reiter, Russel, 54

resistance training, metabolism and, 97–98

Reviva Labs, 106–7

    Carrot Oil Mask, 106

    Green Papaya Hydrogen Peroxide Facial Mask, 106–7

    Light Skin Peel, 106

    Optimum Antioxidant Facial Mask, 43, 106

Rockefeller, Nelson, 121–22

Rogers, Carl, 127

rosemary, 147

Rosenstein, Donald L., 154

sage, 147

salads, blended, 130–31

sauerkraut, 70

saunas

    artificially induced fever and, 114

    dry-air versus wet steam, 112–13

    in Finland, 111–12

    therapeutic benefits of, 113

Save Your Hearing Now (Seidman), 122

savoy cabbage, 50

Schort, Nancy S., iii

Schweitzer, Albert, 5, 18

scurvy, 69–70

sea salt, 163–64

seaweeds, 167

Seidman, Michael D.: *Save Your Hearing Now,* 122

service to others, 18

Seuss, Dr., 217

Shakespeare, William, 18

Shaw, George Bernard, 111

Shazzie: *Detox Your World,* 107

silymarin, 43

simple pleasures, enjoying, 209

skin

    aloe vera and, 39

    alpha lipoic acid and, 59

    artichokes and, 43

    beautifying steps for, 104–7

    brushing of, 107–9

    care products for, 106–7

    diet and, 105

    evening primrose and, 66–67

    exercise and, 105

    functions of, 104

    lavender and, 149

    nature of, 103–4

    papayas and, 156

    positive attitude, meditation and, 106

    sleep and, 105

    vitamin C and, 105

    watercress and, 168

    water, drinking of and, 105

    See also Radiant Health at a Glance Table

sleep

    eating and, 93–94

    lack of, health problems and, 90–91

    melatonin and, 93

    naps and, 92

    need for, 28, 90

    relationships and, 29

    tarragon and, 146

    temperature and, 93

    traffic accidents and, 91

    weight loss and, 28–29, 90

Smith, June B., 229

smoothies, salubrious, 131–33

    60-Second Almond Milk recipe, 195

    Almond Nut Milk recipe, 195

    Apple-Berry-Sunflower-Seed Green Sprouts-Kale recipe, 183

    Apple Green recipe, 186

    Apple-Kale-Lemon recipe, 134

    Apricot-Plum Green recipe, 188

    Berry Green recipe, 184

    Blueberry-Celery-Romaine recipe, 183

    Blueberry Green recipe, 190

    Bosc Pear-Raspberry-Kale recipe, 183

    Carrot-Apple Green recipe, 192

    Citrus Green recipe, 188

    Coconut Green recipe, 192

    Detox Green recipe, 190

    flavor enhancers, supplements for, 181

    Fresh Fig-Kiwi Green recipe, 194

    Fresh Peachy Green Lemonade recipe, 193

    fruits for, 180

    Fruity Green recipe, 187

    ingredients for, 180–81

    Kiwi-Apricot Green recipe, 189

    Kiwi-Banana-Celery recipe, 134

    leafy greens and other vegetables for, 180

    liquids and juices for, 180–81

    Mango Green recipe, 184

    Mango-Parsley recipe, 182

    Nut-Nog Green recipe, 194–95

    Orange-Berry Green recipe, 189

overview of, 179–80
Papaya Green recipe, 187
Peach-Berry Green recipe, 191
Peach-Spinach recipe, 182
Pear-Kale-Mint recipe, 182
Persimmon Green recipe, 186
pineapple and, 158
Pink & Green Lemonade recipe, 193
Prune Green recipe, 185
Purple Green recipe, 192–93
Raspberry Green recipe, 190
Strawberry-Banana-Romaine
    recipe, 134
Sunny's Luscious Sweet Green
    recipe, 194
Sunshine recipe, 185
sweeteners for, 181
thickeners for, 180–81
Tropical Green recipe, 191
V-8 Green recipe, 185–86
snap beans. See green beans
solitude, 122–23, 208
Bible and, 123
Gandhi and, 123
Jesus and, 123
versus loneliness, 123
marriage and, 124
Saint John of the Cross and, 123
vision quests and, 124
Spiegel, Karine, 91–92
spirit, nourishing of, 210
squash, 164–65
Stoddard, Alexandra, iv
Stoner, Gary, 47
stress
breathing and, 77–78
meditation and, 100–102
sleep and, 89

stroke
blackberries and, 47
cherries and, 54
collards and, 59
evening primrose and, 67
grapes and, 142
mangoes and, 152
obesity and, 95
wakame and, 167
sulforaphane, 50
Sun Chlorella, 56
Super Organic Rainbow Salad, 109
Surefire Steps, 14, 16–19
SusanSmithJones.com, 221

tarragon. See French tarragon
Thermal Life® Far Infrared Sauna, 114–15
Thoreau, Henry David, 195
thyrotropin, 91
Tillich, Paul: Courage to Be, 123
turmeric, 147–48
turnips, 165–66
Twain, Mark, 51, 52

ulcers
açai berries and, 38
aloe vera and, 39
cabbage and, 50
meditation and, 101
wheatgrass and, 169
vegetable blossoms, 73
Vegetable Soup/The Fruit Bowl
    (Jones, Warren), 35
vision
apricots and, 41
chicory and, 55
See also Radiant Health at
    a Glance Table

vitamin A
    apricots and, 41
    arugula and, 44
    cherries and, 54
    chicory and, 55
    corn and, 60
    lentils and, 150
    squash and, 165
    watercress and, 168
vitamin C
    limes and, 151
    mangoes and, 152
    Meyer lemons and, 153
    papayas and, 155–56
    plums, prunes and, 159
    skin and, 105
    turnips and, 166
vitamin D, 104
In Vivo, 167
Wachler, Brian S. Boxer, i
wakame, 167–68
watercress, 168–69
water, drinking of, metabolism and,
    99–100
Websites for Susan Smith Jones, 221
weight loss
    blueberries and, 47
    jicama and, 148
    sleep and, 90
    See also fat loss steps; Radiant
    Health at a Glance Table
Weil, Andrew, 84, 164
wheatgrass, 169
White Eagle, 77, 210
    Quiet Mind, 123
whole plant foods, 22
Wild Fermentation (Katz), 70
Winfrey, Oprah, 231

Wired to Meditate (Jones), 12, 93, 102
Wordsworth, William, 125

yellow split peas, 170
Yogananda, Paramahansa, 121

ABOUT THE AUTHOR

"The more you love, the more you're loved,
and the lovelier you are."

— JUNE B. SMITH (SUSAN'S MOM)

For a woman with three of America's most ordinary names, **Susan Smith Jones, M.S., Ph.D.**, certainly has made extraordinary contributions in the fields of optimum holistic health, fitness, nutrition, longevity, and human potential. Selected as one of ten "Healthy American Fitness Leaders" by the President's Council on Physical Fitness & Sports (previous winners include Lance Armstrong, John Wooden, Kathy Smith, Denise Austin, and Richard Simmons), Susan is an award-winning writer and advice columnist. She has authored hundreds of magazine articles, numerous audio programs, and 17 books, including *Choose to Live Fully, BE HEALTHY~STAY BALANCED, Choose to Live Peacefully, Wired to Meditate, Vegetable Soup/The Fruit Bowl* (co-authored with Dianne Warren—for children ages one to ten), *Celebrate Life!, EVERYDAY HEALTH—Pure & Simple, Choose to Be Healthy, The Healing Power of NATUREFOODS,* and *Recipes for HEALTH BLISS: Using NatureFoods to Rejuvenate Your Body & Life* (available from Hay House, June 2009).

Susan appears regularly in the pages and on the covers of national and international publications and is a frequent guest on radio and television talk shows around the country. For 30 years, she taught students, staff, and faculty at UCLA how to be healthy and fit. On her frequent lecture tours, she discusses how to look younger and live longer; boost immunity and energy; minimize stress and maximize joy; prevent and alleviate disease; use food as medicine; set up a healthful kitchen; create meals that rejuvenate the body; detoxify the body with whole foods and fresh juices; make tasty blender meals in seconds; raise healthy children; and bring a sacred balance into your body and life.

An acclaimed holistic health and lifestyle coach, private culinary instructor, and private natural foods chef, Susan works with discerning clients around the world. She creates menus and rejuvenation programs designed to support and complement the needs of her individual clients, as well as the participants at her specialized holistic health retreats. In addition, she serves as a recipe developer and new-product consultant for the health industry.

Susan's inspiring message and innovative techniques for achieving total health in body, mind, and spirit have won her a grateful and enthusiastic following and have put her in constant demand internationally as a health and fitness consultant and motivational speaker (lectures, workshops, and keynote presentations) for community, corporate, and religious/spiritual groups. She also is founder and president of Health Unlimited, a Los Angeles–based consulting firm dedicated to the advancement of peaceful, balanced living and health education. (See Website below for more information about scheduling workshops and appearances.)

Many years ago, when a devastating car accident fractured Susan's back so severely that doctors told her she would never again be physically active and would live a life of chronic pain, she proved them wrong. Her miraculous recovery proved to her that we all have within ourselves everything we need to live our lives to the fullest. She now regularly participates in a variety of fitness activities, including hiking, weight training, in-line skating, biking, Pilates, horseback riding, and yoga. A gifted teacher, Susan brings together modern research and ageless wisdom in all of her work. She resides in Brentwood, Los Angeles.

To receive a special gift (an empowering and heartwarming 77-minute interview with Susan); to find out more about her work, life, and passions; to listen to her telephone seminars from anywhere in the world; or to order any of her book and audio programs easily, please visit: **www.PagingSusan.com**.

❋ ❋ ❋

"Loving yourself is your magical wand."

— LOUISE L. HAY

"If you look at what you have in life,
you'll always have more.
If you look at what you don't have,
you'll never have enough."

— OPRAH WINFREY

"The best way for us to keep fit and healthy
is to watch what we eat and think.
Our choices of thoughts and food are the major parts
of either poor health or good health.
Life has given us unlimited choices,
and it's up to us to educate ourselves
on what really works for us."

— LOUISE L. HAY

"Sometimes you can't see yourself clearly
until you see yourself through the eyes of others."

— ELLEN DEGENERES

HAY HOUSE TITLES OF RELATED INTEREST

YOU CAN HEAL YOUR LIFE, the movie, starring Louise L. Hay & Friends
(available as a 1-DVD program and an expanded 2-DVD set)
Watch the trailer at: **www.LouiseHayMovie.com**

❧ ❧ ❧

The Detox Kit, by Jane Alexander

Everything You Need to Know to Feel Go(o)d,
by Candace Pert, Ph.D., with Nancy Marriott

Home Spa: Creating Your Own Spa Experience with Aromatherapy,
by Judith White

Inner Peace for Busy People: 52 Simple Strategies for Transforming Your Life,
by Joan Borysenko, Ph.D.

Managing People . . . What's Personality Got to Do with It?
by Carol Ritberger, Ph.D.

The Natural Nutrition No-Cook Book: Delicious Food for YOU . . . and Your PETS!
by Kymythy R. Schultze

SHAPE Magazine's Ultimate Body Book:
4 Weeks to Your Best Abs, Butt, Thighs, and More!
by Linda Shelton, with Angela Hynes

Vegetarian Meals for People-on-the-Go: 101 Quick & Easy Recipes,
by Vimala Rodgers

Wheat-Free, Worry-Free: The Art of Happy, Healthy, Gluten-Free Living,
by Danna Korn

You Can Heal Your Life, by Louise L. Hay

❧ ❧ ❧

All of the above are available at your local bookstore,
or may be ordered by contacting Hay House (see last page).

❧ ❧ ❧

We hope you enjoyed this Hay House book.
If you'd like to receive a free catalog featuring additional Hay House books and products,
or if you'd like information about the Hay Foundation, please contact:

Hay House, Inc.
P.O. Box 5100
Carlsbad, CA 92018-5100

(760) 431-7695 or (800) 654-5126
(760) 431-6948 (fax) or (800) 650-5115 (fax)
www.hayhouse.com® • www.hayfoundation.org

Published and distributed in Australia by: Hay House Australia Pty. Ltd.,
18/36 Ralph St., Alexandria NSW 2015 • *Phone:* 612-9669-4299 • *Fax:* 612-9669-4144
www.hayhouse.com.au

Published and distributed in the United Kingdom by: Hay House UK, Ltd., 292B Kensal Rd.,
London W10 5BE • *Phone:* 44-20-8962-1230 • *Fax:* 44-20-8962-1239
www.hayhouse.co.uk

Published and distributed in the Republic of South Africa by: Hay House SA (Pty), Ltd.,
P.O. Box 990, Witkoppen 2068 • *Phone/Fax:* 27-11-467-8904
orders@psdprom.co.za • www.hayhouse.co.za

Published in India by: Hay House Publishers India, Muskaan Complex, Plot No. 3,
B-2, Vasant Kunj, New Delhi 110 070 • *Phone:* 91-11-4176-1620 • *Fax:* 91-11-4176-1630
www.hayhouse.co.in

Distributed in Canada by: Raincoast, 9050 Shaughnessy St.,
Vancouver, B.C. V6P 6E5 • *Phone:* (604) 323-7100 • *Fax:* (604) 323-2600
www.raincoast.com

Tune in to **HayHouseRadio.com**® for the best in inspirational talk radio featuring
top Hay House authors! And, sign up via the Hay House USA Website to receive the
Hay House online newsletter and stay informed about what's going on with your favorite authors.
You'll receive bimonthly announcements about Discounts and Offers, Special Events,
Product Highlights, Free Excerpts, Giveaways, and more!
www.hayhouse.com®

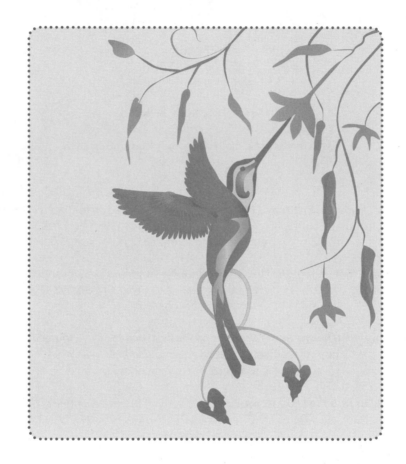